RadTool Nuclear Medicine Flash Facts

Bital Savir-Baruch • Bruce J. Barron

RadTool Nuclear Medicine Flash Facts

Illustrations by
Eric Jablonowski

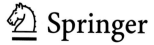

Bital Savir-Baruch
Loyola University Medical Center
Maywood
Illinois
USA

Bruce J. Barron
School of Medicine
Emory University
Atlanta
USA

Illustrations by

Eric Jablonowski
School of Medicine
Emory University
Atlanta
USA

ISBN 978-3-319-24634-5   ISBN 978-3-319-24636-9   (eBook)
DOI 10.1007/978-3-319-24636-9

Library of Congress Control Number: 2016941755

© Springer International Publishing Switzerland 2017
This work is subject to copyright. All rights are reserved by the Publisher, whether the whole or part of the material is concerned, specifically the rights of translation, reprinting, reuse of illustrations, recitation, broadcasting, reproduction on microfilms or in any other physical way, and transmission or information storage and retrieval, electronic adaptation, computer software, or by similar or dissimilar methodology now known or hereafter developed.
The use of general descriptive names, registered names, trademarks, service marks, etc. in this publication does not imply, even in the absence of a specific statement, that such names are exempt from the relevant protective laws and regulations and therefore free for general use.
The publisher, the authors and the editors are safe to assume that the advice and information in this book are believed to be true and accurate at the date of publication. Neither the publisher nor the authors or the editors give a warranty, express or implied, with respect to the material contained herein or for any errors or omissions that may have been made.

Printed on acid-free paper

This Springer imprint is published by Springer Nature
The registered company is Springer International Publishing AG Switzerland

Preface

Nuclear medicine includes sophisticated imaging technology. It encompasses a complex integration of physics, chemistry, radiation safety, physiology, pathophysiology, pathology, histology, radiology, internal medicine, endocrinology, hematology, radiation oncology, cardiology, and other disciplines in the form of a single image. Each radiotracer has a specific distribution which may result in an identifiable imaging characteristic. The same radiotracer can be tailored for different clinical indications by changing the route of administration and sequence of imaging. Understanding the mechanism, distribution, and clearance of radiotracers may be challenging.

This book offers a unique summary of facts in nuclear medicine associated with colorful illustrations and variety of images to allow for:

- Fast learning of physical, chemical characteristics and distribution of each commonly used radiotracer and radiopharmaceuticals.
- Recalling essential facts for each radiopharmaceutical that may be used in everyday practice by radiologists and nuclear medicine physicians, residents, and students in training and for board examinations (as flash cards).
- Identification of patterns of abnormal tracer distribution to allow narrowed differential diagnosis.

Maywood, IL, USA   Bital Savir-Baruch
Atlanta, GA, USA   Bruce J. Barron

Flash Fact Recommended Schedule for Your Boards (From the Authors' Point of View)

Use 2.5 months for studying, assuming you will use 2–4 h a day to study.

Learn while in residency and prepare for the in-service exams as if it is "the" board exam. Hopefully by the end of your training, you already reviewed the suggested list or a similar list at least once. Additional suggested reading while in training is the package insert of each radiopharmaceutical.

Step 1 – Start with *The Requisites: Nuclear Medicine*, by Harvey A. Ziessman. Use this book as your baseline. As needed, use *Essentials of Nuclear Medicine* by Fred A. Mettler for additional information. Reviewing the images from both books is essential.

Step 2 – *Case-Based Nuclear Medicine* by Kevin J. Donohoe et al.

Step 3 – "*Radcases Nuclear Medicine*" by Daniel Appelbaum et al. – Rad Case book you should use it as interactive practice online on the RadCases website.

Step 4 – *Nuclear Medicine: Case Review Series*, by Harvey A. Ziessman et al.

Step 5 – Cardiac books; read one book of your choice and use the other for images only.

Nuclear Cardiology Review by Wael A. Jaber et al.

Atlas of Nuclear Cardiology by Ami E. Iskandrian et al.

Step 6 – Physics: *Essentials of Nuclear Medicine Physics and Instrumentations* by Rachel A. Powsner et al. Read it all.

Step 7 – Pediatrics: *Pediatric Nuclear Medicine* by S.T. Treves; use this book for images and fast reading. Review all images in this book.

Step 8 – Now focus on practicing what you learned:

RadTool Nuclear Medicine Flash Facts By Savir-Baruch et al.

RadPrimer NM questions.

Nuclear Medicine Board Review: Questions and Answers for Self-Assessment by C. Goldfarb et al.

Look at EKG strips to recognize LBBB, 2nd- and 3rd-degree heart block. Review the cardiac protocols and indications (use EKG flash facts).

Step 9 – At the end, review cases you marked while studying.

Please note we have no financial interest in any of the books or suggested reading materials listed above except this book.

Good Luck.

Acknowledgments

We would like to thank the following colleagues who helped us in the preparation of this book:

Raghuveer K Halkar, MD, who shared with us multiple key images in nuclear medicine; Nicholas A Plaxton, MD, and Valeria M Moncayo, MD, for their contribution to this book at its early stages by collecting and presenting facts on radiopharmaceuticals while in residency; Fabio Esteves, MD, for sharing his cardiac image collection; Chad G Morsch, BS, CEP, for sharing his EKG strips collection; Kathleen E Detwiler PhD, MD, who typed our handwritten radiation safety notes into a word document; Robert H Wagner, MD, for his support in time and spirit; and Medhat Sam Gabriel, MD, and Stephen Karesh, PhD, for spending their free time reviewing and editing this book, page by page, line by line, prior to submission.

Bital Savir-Baruch, MD
Bruce J. Barron, MD, MHA, FACNM
Eric Jablonowski, AS

I would like to thank Bruce J Barron, MD, MHA, FACNM, for joining me in the book preparation and sharing in this book his unique collection of images. I would like to thank Eric Jablonowski for working around the clock while sharing his great talent as the illustrator of this book. The book wouldn't be the same without his personal touch. A special acknowledgment goes to my mentors in the Residency Program at Emory University Hospital: Raghuveer K Halkar, MD, and David M Schuster, MD. I am the physician I am due to my great educators. And thanks also to my colleagues at Loyola University Medical Center: Robert H Wagner, MD; Medhat Sam Gabriel, MD; James R Halama, PhD; Stephen Karesh, PhD; and Davide Bova, MD, for their support.

Last and most important, I would like to thank my beloved husband Amos and our two boys Liam and Ely as well as my parents Yossi and Livna, who dedicated their time and effort to support me in my long path; I couldn't have made it without them.

With love,
Bital Savir-Baruch, MD

Contents

List of Contributors

We would like to thank the following colleagues who helped us in the preparation of this book:

Contributors

Tina M. Buehner, MS, CNMT, RT   Department of Radiology, Loyola University Health System/Gottlieb Memorial Hospital, Maywood, IL, USA

Kathleen E. Detwiler, PhD, MD   Department of Radiology, Loyola University Medical Center, Maywood, IL, USA

Fabio Esteves, MD   Department of Radiology and Molecular Imaging, Emory University Hospital, Atlanta, GA, USA

Medhat Sam Gabriel, MD   Department of Radiology, Loyola University Medical Center, Maywood, IL, USA

Raghuveer K. Halkar, MD Department of Radiology and Molecular Imaging, Emory University Hospital, Atlanta, GA, USA

Stephen Karesh, PhD   Department of Radiology, Loyola University Medical Center, Maywood, IL, USA

Valeria M. Moncayo, MD   Department of Radiology and Molecular Imaging, Emory University Hospital, Atlanta, GA, USA

Nicholas A. Plaxton, MD   Department of Nuclear Medicine, Bay Pines Veterans Affairs Hospital, Bay Pine, FL, USA

Ila Sethi, MD   Department of Radiology and Molecular Imaging, Emory University Hospital, Atlanta, GA, USA

Robert H. Wagner, MD   Department of Radiology, Loyola University Medical Center, Maywood, IL, USA

Coauthor

Flash Facts Radiation Biology; Flash Facts Photon Interaction with Matter; Flash
   Facts Interaction of Charged Particles with Atoms in Matter, Detectors, Collimators

James R. Halama, PhD   Department of Radiology, Loyola University Medical
   Center, Maywood, IL, USA

Flash Facts Equipment, Quality Control; Flash Facts Radiation Safety, Radionuclide
   Decay; Flash Facts Radiation Biology

Stephen Karesh, PhD   Department of Radiology, Loyola University Medical
   Center, Maywood, IL, USA

EKG

Chad G. Morsch, BS, CEP   Department of Radiology, Loyola University Medical
   Center, Maywood, IL, USA

Dacryoscintigraphy

David C. Brandon, MD   Department of Radiology and Molecular Imaging,
   Emory University Hospital, Atlanta, GA, USA and the Department of Nuclear
   Medicine, Atlanta Veterans Affairs Medical Center, Atlanta, GA, USA

MPI

Greg Gregory Wegenast, PA-C   Department of Nuclear Medicine, Atlanta
   Veterans Affairs Medical Center, Atlanta, GA, USA

Part 1: Basics of Nuclear Medicine Flash Facts

Contents

© Springer International Publishing Switzerland 2017
B. Savir-Baruch, B.J. Barron, *RadTool Nuclear Medicine Flash Facts*,
DOI 10.1007/978-3-319-24636-9_1

1   Flash Facts Radiation Safety

1 rem = 1000 mrem = 10 mSv = 0.01 Sv

Radiation Exposure
- Public exposure: 100 mrem/year = 0.1 rem/year = 1 mSv/year = 0.001 Sv/year.
- Occupational exposure: 5,000 mrem/year = 5 rem/year = 50 mSv/year = 0.05 Sv/year.
- Pregnancy exposure: 0.5 rem = 500 mrem = 5 mSv from date of conception until end of pregnancy (10 CFR Part 35.1208).
- Radiation area exposure: > 5 mrem/h at 30 cm.
- High radiation area: > 0.1 rem/h at 30 cm. Door sign: Yellow color for high radiation area, which requires RWP (radiation work permit) for entry. Example of a door sign: "Dose rate at this point is (x) mrem/h, posted on (Date) by (radiation personnel)."
- Public area radiation level limits (unrestricted area): 100 mrem in 1 year and 2 mrem in any 1 h.
- Patient release after I-131 treatment:
  <7 mrem/h at 1 m from the chest or <33 mCi I-131 NaI (NRC Regulations).
  <5 mrem/h at 1 m from the chest or <30 mCi I-131 NaI (some Agreement State Regulations).
- Body exposure:
  Eye limit dose (lens): 15 rem = 0.15 Sv = 150 mSv = 0.15 Sv/year.
  Whole body (same as occupational exposure): 5 rem = 0.05 Sv = 50 mSv.
  Extremity dose: 50 rem = 0.5 Sv = 500 mSv.
- Household contact exposure: < 0.5 rem (5 mSv); child < 0.1 rem (1 mSv).
- Yellow radiation sign: Caution radiation area; personnel dosimetry required.

Written Directive required for   30 μCi I-131 or 1.11MBq.

Disposal of Radioactive Material
1. Monitor surface of each container.
2. Survey surface with Geiger counter, < 0.05 mrem/h.
3. Remove shields to measure properly.
4. Remove labeling.
5. Record day collected and disposal data.

Minor Spill (Major Spill Is Above These Values)
Tl-201, Tc-99m <100 mCi.
I-131 < 1 mCi.
I-123, In-111, Ga-67 < 10 mCi.

Procedure for Minor Spills
1. Stop work, and evacuate all personals.
2. Use gloves.
3. Absorbent paper and label with "Caution Radiation Material."
4. Transfer to radiation waste.
5. Survey (continue to clean until no counts are detected using Geiger counter).
6. Survey body (clothing, shoes, gloves etc.).
7. Report to radiation safety officer (RSO).

Major Spills Call RSO.

Medical Event (NRC 10 CFR Part 35.3045)

- Definition: An event takes place upon administration of wrong dose (not within ±20 % of prescribed dose; some states or institutions require ±10 % with therapeutic agents); wrong radiotracer, wrong route of administration, wrong patient, wrong treatment, and leaking seal source.
- Reportable event: Administration resulting in whole-body exposure of >0.05 Sv (5 rem) effective dose equivalent or 0.5 Sv (50 rem) to an organ or tissue and skin. Must be reported by telephone call within 24 h and notified in writing within 15 days.
- Recordable event: Administration resulting in whole-body exposure of <0.05 Sv (5 rem) effective dose equivalent and 0.5 Sv (50 rem) to an organ or tissue and skin.

Package Safety and Unpacking

1. Must unpack radioactive shipments within 3 h of receipt.
2. Survey surface with Geiger–Muller counter.
3. Wipe test 100 cm^2 of box surface.
4. Remove vial containing the radiopharmaceutical.

Radioactive Labels

- White I <0.5 mrem/h at 1 m.
- Yellow II < 50 mrem/h at surface.
- <1 mrem/h at 1 m.
- Yellow III < 200 mrem/h at surface.
- <10 mrem/h at 1 m.

Breast-Feeding Guidelines*

- I-131 *and* Ga-67 – For I-131, complete cessation of breast-feeding for this child.
- Avoid Ga-67 scan on a breast-feeding patient due to high breast radiation dose.
- I-123 (cyclotron produced therefore not contaminated with I-124): Pump and dump for 48 h.
- Tl-201: Pump and dump for 96 h.
- Tc-99m: Pump and dump for 12 h (Tc-99m pertechnetate, 4 h only).

Suggested Reading

- Code of Federal Regulations Title 10 Part 35 at http://www.nrc.gov/reading-rm/doc-collections/cfr/part035
- *Nuclear Medicine: The requisites 4th edition By Harvey A Ziessman MD

2   Radionuclide Decay

X = element name
A = atomic mass (number of protons + neutrons)
Z = number of protons

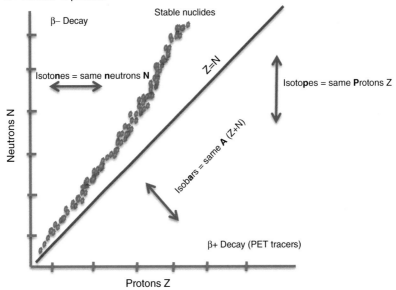

Radionuclide decay graph

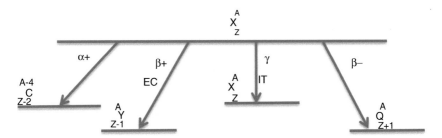

Radionuclide decay scheme. *EC* electron capture, *IT* isomeric transition (originated from the nucleus)

Radionuclide decay table

Tracer	Half-life	Production	Decay	g-ray E (Kev)
Co-57	270.9 days	Cyclotron	EC	122 (85.6 %)
F-18	109.8 min	Cyclotron	β+	511
Ga-67	78.3 h	Cyclotron	EC	91 (3.6 %) 185 (23.5 %) 300 (4.4 %) 394 (4.4 %)
In-111	2.8 days	Cyclotron	EC	172 (89.6 %) 247 (94 %)
I-123	13.2 h	Cyclotron	EC	159 (83.0 %)
I-125	60 days	Nuclear reactor	EC	35 (7 %)
I-131	8 days	Nuclear reactor	β–	364 (81.8 %)
Mo-99	66 h	Nuclear reactor	β–	740 (13.6 %) 778 (4.7 %)
N-13	10 min	Cyclotron	β+	511
0–15	2 s	Cyclotron	β+	511
P-32	14.3 days	Nuclear reactor	β–	None
Rb-82	76 s	^{82}Sr. generator	β+ EC	511 776 (15 %) – prompt gamma
Sm-153	47 h	Nuclear reactor	β–, γ	103 (28 %)
Sr-89	50.5 days	Nuclear reactor	β–	None
Tc-99m	6 h	^{99}Mo generator	IT	140
Tl-201	73.5 h	Cyclotron	EC	Mercury X-ray 69–80
Xenon-131	5.2 days	Nuclear reactor	β–	81 (36.6 %)
Y-90	64.5 h	Nuclear reactor	β-	Bremsstrahlung (X-rays)
Ra-223	11.4 days	Decay of uranium-235	α	None

3   Flash Facts: Radiation Biology

Units
- R = roentgen = gamma- or X-ray radiation in air (not tissue).
- REM = Roentgen equivalent man = normalized radiation dose in a tissue to account for biological effects.
- 1 g-ray = 1 J/kg tissue (absorbed) = 100 rad.
- Q = radiation type weighting factors; photons, electrons, betas, and positrons, Q = 1; protons > 2 MeV, Q = 5; neutrons, Q = 5–10; alpha particles, Q = 20.
- W = organ tissue weighting factors summed over all exposed organs to compute an REM or effective dose in sievert

Cell Cycle Sensitivity S < G1 < G2 < M.

Oxygen-Enhancing Ratio (OER) Enhancing of radiation damage by adding O_2 to the matrix.

LD 50/30 Lethal dose required to kill 50 % of population in 30 day. Humans' lethal dose is measured in 60 days. LD 50/60 = 3–5 Gy for human.

Stochastic Effect Probability that radiation will cause damage = dose dependent

Nonstochastic (Deterministic) Describe cause and effect relationships between radiation and damage. Have a threshold below which has no side effect. Once threshold is crossed, diseases will develop (2 Gy to eye = cataract).

Basic Science Formulas

Half life, $T_{1/2} = 0.693 / \lambda$

Effective half life $= 1 / T_e = 1 / T_p + 1 / T_b$ Or

$$T_e = \left(T_b \times T_p\right) / \left(T_p + T_b\right) \mathrm{p} = \text{physical}, \mathrm{b} = \text{biological}$$

Decay constant $= \lambda = 0.693 / T_{1/2}$

Decay equation $= A_t = A_o \times 0.5^{(t/t_{1/2})}$ Or $A(t) = A(0) \times e^{-\lambda t}$ $\left(\mathrm{t} = \text{elapsed time}\right)$

Suggested Reading
- NRC.ORG
- Zanzonico P (2008) Routine quality control of clinical nuclear medicine instrumentation: a brief review. J Nucl Med 49(7):1114–1131. doi:10.2967/jnumed.107.050203.
- https://www.aur.org/uploadedFiles/Meeting/pdf/NRCRegulations2008.pdf

4   Flash Facts: Photon Interaction with Matter

Mechanism Photon energy will be moving in space and will interact with atoms. Types of interactions will be determined by the atomic number of the absorbed atom and by the energy of the photon. Most common energies used in nuclear medicine are in the range of 71–511 KeV (Tl-201 to PET agents).

Compton scatter Radiation interaction with low-atomic-number materials in lower energies (most common in low KeV energy medical fields). Partial photon energy is transferred to an outer shell electron. Loss of electron from the outer shell (More frequently seen and associated with Compton Scattered reaction) → unbound electron will fill the vacancy.

Photoelectric effect Radiation interaction with high atomic numbers. Photon energy quantitatively transferred to the inner shell electron. Outer shell electron will fill the vacancy → X-ray released. For example, lead interaction with lower KeV energies will result in X-rays and photoelectric effect.

Pair production Interaction of high-energy photon (E > 1020 KeV) with matter. Produces positron and electron. The positron annihilates a different electron and annihilation radiation is produced. 2 photons, 511 keV, 180° apart.

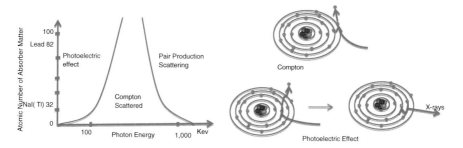

Calculating Energy Loss Due to Attenuation

$$I_{out} = I_{in} \times 0.5^{(\text{thickness}/\text{HVL})} \text{ or } I_{out} = I_{in} \times e^{-\mu x}$$

μ = linear attenuation coefficient (constant for each material).

Half-Value Layer (HVL) Thickness of attenuator required to reduce beam intensity to half its original value.

Tenth-Value Layer (TVL) Thickness of attenuator required to reduce beam intensity to one tenth its original value (for Tc = 99 in lead, HVL = 0.017 cm (50 %); TVL = 0.083 cm (10 %)).

Linear Energy Transfer (LET) Fraction of energy deposited in a given distance by the charged particle or photon moving through matter.

5   Flash Facts: Interaction of Charged Particles with Atoms in Matter

Excitation (No Loss of Electron)
Energy enough to move inner shell electron to other shell electron → electron from outer shell will replace the vacant space ("musical chairs") → characteristic X-rays.

Ionization (Loss of Electron)
Loss of electron from the inner shell (less frequently seen and associated with photoelectric reaction) → electron from outer shell will replace the vacant space → characteristic X-rays.

Loss of electron from the outer shell (more frequently seen and associated with Compton scattered reaction) → unbound electron will fill the vacant space.

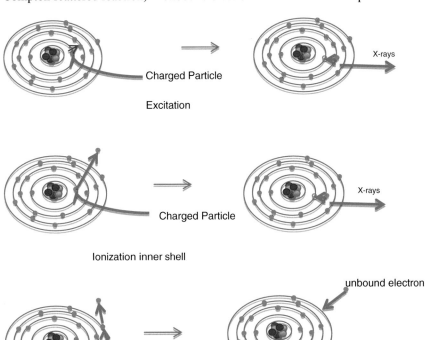

Charged Particle

X-rays

Excitation

Charged Particle

X-rays

Ionization inner shell

unbound electron

Charged Particle

Ionization outer shell

Annihilation (Interaction of β⁺ Particle with Electron)

Unstable elements undergoing positron emission release β⁺ particle [Positron → Neutron + β⁺+ V (neutrino)]. β⁺ particle will interact with electron to form annihilation → Release of two perpendicular 511 KeV gamma photons.

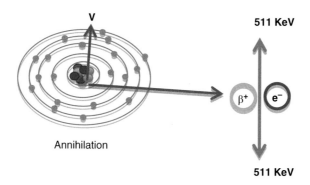

Bremsstrahlung

The release of x-rays photons after small charged particles (such as β⁺, β⁻) passed near the nucleus of atoms in matter.

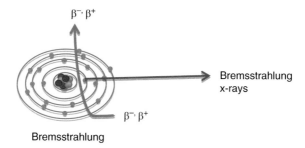

6   Flash Facts: Detectors

Gas Field Detectors
- Iodination chambers: Rate of ionization is proportional to the energy coming from the radiotracer in the chamber.
- Dose calibration: Optimal geometric efficacy. Cannot separate between types of energies – only determine the radiation dose.
- Survey meter: Measures at mR/Hr (use to determine exposed I-131 dose).
- Pocket dosimeter: Measures exposure to photon over time.
- Proportional counters: Can separate types of energies.
- Proportional survey meter: Use to distinguish types of energies including alpha radiation.
- Geiger counter: Geiger–Muller – Chamber filled with argon (halogen or methane) gas to allow increased voltage. Cannot separate between types of energy.
- Photographic detectors: Film badge.

Semiconductors
- Cadmium Zinc Telluride (CdZnTe), Cadmium Telluride (CdTe), Zinc Telluride.
- High density semiconductors – Direct energy conversion Photon $\rightarrow$ semiconductor $\rightarrow$ electron $\rightarrow$ signal.

Scintillation Detectors
- Thyroid Probe, Well counter (good geometric efficacy), Gamma camera. Indirect conversion of radiation energy $\rightarrow$ light $\rightarrow$ electron.
- Structure and mechanism: Gamma ray/X-ray $\rightarrow$ NaI crystal $\rightarrow$ Photomultiplier tube (every 1 Kev gamma ray $\rightarrow$ 40 light photon) $\rightarrow$ preamplifiers $\rightarrow$ amplifiers $\rightarrow$ pulse -height analyzer (define the energy window to accept the needed level of energy) $\rightarrow$ signal.

Semiconductors vs. scintillation detectors

	CZT	NaI
Signal conversion	Direct	Indirect
Temperature	Room temperature	Requires cold environment
Atomic number	+++	++
Energy resolution	<4 %	>10 %
Size	+	+++
Cost	+++	+

PET Detector Crystals
- *Density* (*greater stopping power*): LYSO/LSO > BGO > GSO > NaI(Tl).
- *Decay time* (*define dead time*): NaI(Tl) > BGO > GSO > LYSO/LSO.
- *Light yield* (*increase energy resolution*): NaI(Tl) > LYSO/LSO > GSO > BGO.

Resolutions
- *Intrinsic resolution* – Ability to localize the interaction of the gamma energy with the crystal.
- *Spatial resolution* – Ability to separate two adjacent dotes (depends on intrinsic and collimator resolutions).
- *Energy resolution* – Ability to separate between different energies.

6.1   Gamma Specific Detectors

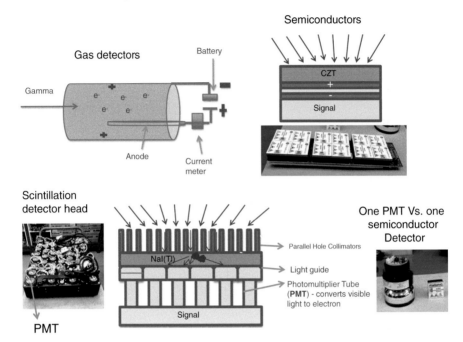

CZT. Manufactured by GE Healthcare. Haifa, Israel

7   Flash Facts: Collimators

Increased length and narrowed collimator bores → increased resolution but decreased sensitivity

- Low energy: Tc-99m, Xe-133, Tl-201.
- Medium energy: In-111, Ga-67, I-123.
- High Energy: I-131.
- Pinhole magnifies small objects, such as thyroid gland and widely used in pediatric population.

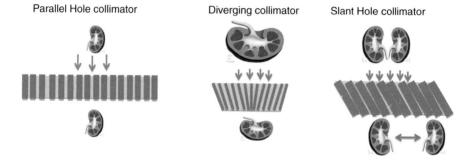

Parallel Hole collimator   Diverging collimator   Slant Hole collimator

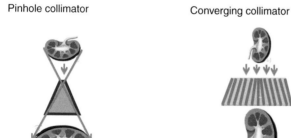

Pinhole collimator   Converging collimator

8   Flash Facts: Equipment Quality Control

Mo-99/Tc-99 Generator Purity

Radionuclide purity: Mo breakthrough <0.15 µCi/ mCi Tc-99m elute at the time of administration. Test: Mo-99 emits 740 and 780 KeV gamma rays; therefore, Mo-99 is assayed first directly in the special lead pig supplied by the manufacturer of your dose calibrator. Tc-99m is then assayed directly in the plastic sleeve. Activity (µCi) of Mo-99 is divided by activity (mCi) of Tc-99m to obtain a ratio. If test is performed in reverse order, failure is extremely likely due to residual charge on ionization chamber that takes a few minutes to dissipate.

Mo–99 Breakthrough Test

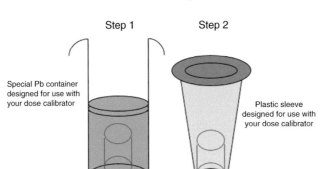

Chemical purity: Al^{3+} ion < 10 µg/mL eluate. Test: colorimetric, qualitative spot. Aluminum ion breakthrough: Al^{3+} ion is measured colorimetrically. A drop of the eluate is placed on one end of a special test paper; a drop of a standard solution of Al^{3+}, concentration 10 ppm, is placed on the other end of the test strip. If the color at the center of the drop of eluate is less red than that of the standard solution, the eluate has passed the Al^{3+} ion breakthrough test. Units may be also be expressed as mg/ml. Diagram at right: test passed.

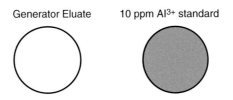

Excess of Al^{3+} in Tc-99m-sulfur colloid → abnormal lung uptake.
Excess Al^{3+} in Tc-99m MDP → abnormal liver uptake.
Radiochemical purity: Tc-99m TcO_4^{1-} is desired product; HR Tc is the impurity. Oxidation state of 4+.
Test: Measured using paper chromatography.

Dose Calibrator

- <u>Daily</u>: *Constancy test.* This test, performed at installation and daily, measures instrument precision and is designed to show that a long-lived source, usually 30 y Cs-137, yields reproducible readings on a daily basis on all isotope settings we are likely to use. The Cs-137 source is placed in the dose calibrator. Activity is then measured on the Cs-137 setting and all other settings used on a daily basis. Values are recorded in the dose calibrator logbook and are compared with recent values to determine if instrument is maintaining constancy on a daily basis.
- <u>Quarterly</u>: *Linearity test.* This test, performed at installation and quarterly, is designed to prove that the dose calibrator readout is linear for sources varying from the µCi range through the µCi range. A high-activity Tc-99m source (50–300 mCi) is measured at T_0 and at predetermined time intervals up to 48 h. Expected and actual measurements are compared (and may be analyzed graphically) to determine if the instrument is linear throughout the activity range we are likely to encounter.
- <u>Annually</u>: *Accuracy test.* This test, performed at installation and annually, is designed to show that the calibrator is giving correct readings throughout the entire energy scale that we are likely to encounter. Low-, medium-, and high-energy standards (usually Co-57, Ba-133 or Cs-137, and Co-60, respectively) are measured in the dose calibrator using appropriate settings. Standard and measured values are compared.
- <u>At installation/after repair</u>: *Geometry test.* This test, performed at installation, is designed to show that correct readings can be obtained regardless of the sample size or geometry. 0.5 ml of Tc-99m in a 10 ml syringe (activity 25 mCi) is measured in the dose calibrator, and the value obtained is recorded. The activity is then diluted with water to 2, 3, 5, and 10 ml. At each of these points, a reading is taken and the value recorded. Data are then evaluated to determine the effect of sample geometry on the dose calibrator reading. If instrument is geometry dependent, it may be necessary to routinely correct readings obtained when using calibrator.
- Deviation from standard or expected values must be within ± 10 %. If deviation >10 %, then obligation is to record value, note repair or recalibration of instrument, retest, and record new values.

Survey Meters

Portable, battery operated, gas filled, ionization detectors used to monitor ambient radiation levels and include:
- Cutie pies used for high-flux fields containing X- or γ-rays (so named because the formula is $Q \times d \times \prod$).
- Geiger-Müller (GM) counters. Have high sensitivity and are used for low-level survey/contamination. Operation is not energy dependent. Signal amplitude is independent of energy.

Quality Control Testing

- Daily

  Battery checks: Performed with a display indicating whether the voltage supplied by the battery is within the acceptable operating range.

  Daily constancy test: Measurement of count rate sensitivity. Measurement is performed with a long-lived source such as Cs-137.

  Daily background count rate: should be measured in an area remote from radioactive sources within the nuclear medicine facility to confirm that the survey meter has not been contaminated.

- Installation, Annually, or after Repair:

  Accuracy calibration: determined using suitable long-lived reference source (typically Cs-137). Value reported in mR/Hr.

Well Counter/Thyroid Probe
Quality Control Testing

- Daily

  Calibrate: Performed with Cs-137 by adjustment of PMT high voltage and amplifier gain so that the Cs-137 gamma photopeak is centered at 662 kev

- Installation, Annual, Repair

  Efficiency (sensitivity): Measured in cpm/Bq. The measured day-to-day exposure or counting rates should be within 10 %; if not, the meter should be recalibrated.

Gamma Camera

- Daily: *Uniformity test.* Acquire image of Tc-99m or Co-57 flood source to ensure *uniformity* in the flood image. Nonuniformity may be due to imbalance of PMT, high voltage and gains, or collimator damage.

- Weekly: Measure *spatial resolution and linearity* with a four-quadrant bar phantom. For spatial resolution, identify the quadrant in the image of the smallest visible bar size. For linearity, the image of the bars should appear straight and not curved or bowed at the camera periphery or around the PMTs.

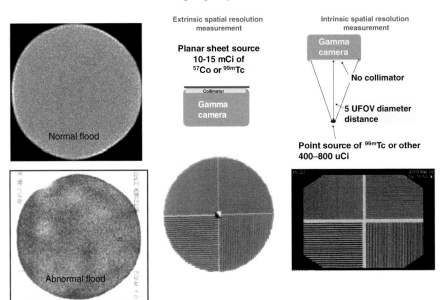

SPECT

<u>Monthly</u>

- *Uniformity calibration*: Performed with a high count flood acquisition for each detector. Obtained with count rate ten times as high as daily flood image (30–100 million counts).

  Unfixed non-uniformities in detector flood images will result in a non-uniform rings like appearance, "bull's-eye", artifact (*blue arrow*).

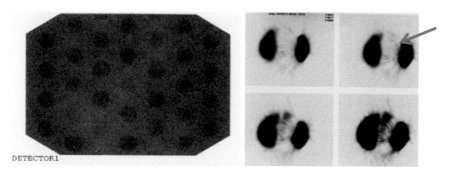

- *Center of rotation (COR)*: Calibration monthly by SPECT imaging of point sources of Tc-99m on imaging pallet. Identifies the center location (centroid) of the point source images seen on all detector viewing angles. Uncorrected COR errors will result in a ring artifact (*red arrow*).

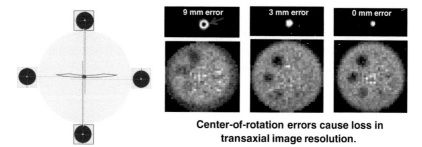

Center-of-rotation errors cause loss in transaxial image resolution.

Suggested Reading

- QC Protocols Gamma Camera & SPECT Systems. James R Halama, PhD. http://www.aapm.org/meetings/amos2/pdf/35-9798-70158-156.pdf

9   Flash Facts: EKG

EKG Lead Positioning (Fig. 1)
- **Precordial leads (V1–V6): V1**, fourth right intercostal space; **V2**, fourth left intercostal space; **V3**, between V2 and V4; **V4**, fifth intercostal space (midclavicular line); **V5**, fifth intercostal space midway between V4 and V6; and **V6**, fifth intercostal space – midaxillary line.
- **Limb leads:** As illustrated in the figure: right arm (RA) and left arm (LA) wrists and right leg (RL) and left leg (LL) ankles.
- *Lateral leads*: I, aVL, V_5, and V_6. *Inferior leads*: II, III, and aVF. *Anterior leads*: V_3 and V_4. *Septal leads*: V_1 and V_2.

Vectors   Vector scheme for the evaluation of axis (Fig. 2). *Instruction*: Look for the most equiphasic lead (R and S are almost equal) → determine if QRS is positive or negative (sum of R and S) → use the vector schema and follow the vector toward the positive or negative direction (if lead is completely equiphasic, this is the axis).
   In case of no equiphasic lead:
- Technique 1 (Fig. 3). Find all the perpendicular vectors (I+aVF, II+aVL, III+aVR) → determine by the EKG trace if the sum of QRS is positive or negative → trace it on the vectors scheme → axis will be approximately the average of the space shared by the three pairs.
- Technique 2 (Fig. 4). Choose one perpendicular vectors (I + aVF or II + aVL or III + aVR). From the EKG, count the numbers of small squares for each vector → On the axis chart, along the chosen pair of vectors count same number of small squares at the positive or negative directions (according to the EKG) → draw a perpendicular line → meeting point of the two lines is the axis.

Normal contraction (Fig. 5)   *P* – atrial depolarization; *QRS* – ventricular depolarization; *T* – ventricular repolarization.

EKG Paper   Each small box is 1 mm or 0.04 s. Each large box is 5 mm or 0.20 s.

Calculating HR (Figs. 6 and 7)   Starting point at the R → moving 5 mm at a time → 300 bpm → 150 → 100 → 75 → 60 → 50 → 43 → 38 bpm. Or 300 divided by the number of large boxes (intervals).

Normal values   PR interval – 0.12–0.20 s. QRS interval – 0.04–0.11 s.

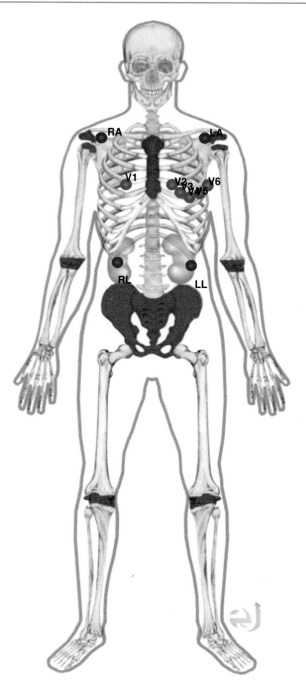

Fig. 1 Position of electrodes

Rhythm

- **Normal sinus rhythm (NSR)** HR 60–100 bpm. *Sinus bradycardia*: <60 bpm. *Sinus tachycardia*: >100 bpm. *Sinus flutter*: >240 bpm. *Sinus fibrillation*: >300 bpm.
- **Sinus arrhythmia** Normal EKG trace with slight rhythm irregularity – normal phenomenon. May be affected by respiration.
- **Arrhythmias with automaticity focus** *Ventricular tachycardia* 100–250 bpm, *flutter* 250–350 bpm, and *fibrillation* 350–450 bpm.
- **Premature atrial contraction (PAC)** An early beat originating in the atria but away from the SA node → P wave is visible however differs from sinus P waves.
- **Paroxysmal supraventricular tachycardia (PSVT)** Narrow QRS complex. HR of 150–250 bpm. No P waves. Treatment with adenosine bolus or cardioversion.
- **Premature ventricular tachycardia (PVC)** QRS duration ≥ must be at least 0.12 s. Isolated PVCs are common in normal patients. > 6 PVC in 1 min is pathological.

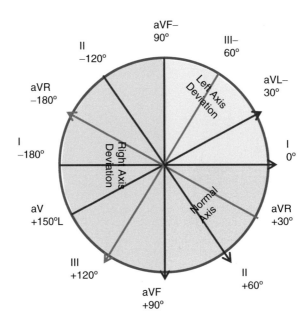

Fig. 2 Axis chart

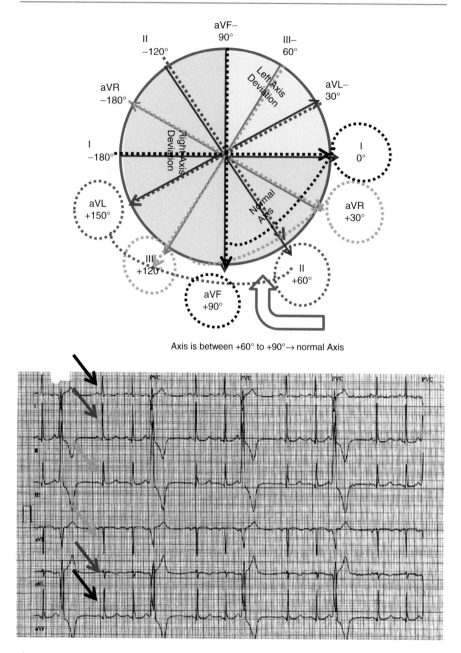

Axis is between +60° to +90°→ normal Axis

Fig. 3 Axis evaluation in EKG without an equiphasic lead. Technique 1

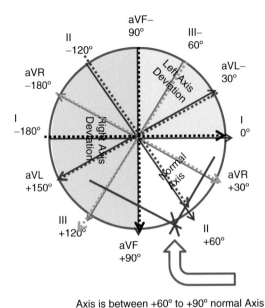

Axis is between +60° to +90° normal Axis

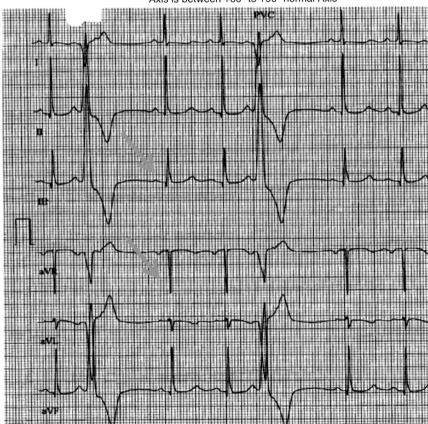

Fig. 4 Axis evaluation in EKG without an equiphasic lead, using only one pair of vectors. Technique 2. Lead III is approximately 13 small squares in the positive direction. Lead AVR is approximately 16 small squares in the negative direction

Fig. 5   P – atrial
depolarization; QRS –
ventricular depolarization;
T – ventricular
repolarization

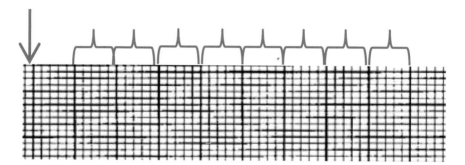

Fig. 6   Heart rate starting point at the R peak moving 5 mm at a time → 300 → 150 → 100 → 75 → 60 → 50 → 43 → 38

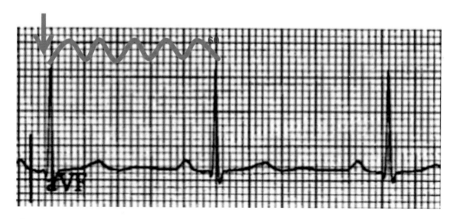

Fig. 7   Example of five large-box intervals with HR of ~60

- **Ventricular bigeminy PVC** Sinus beat follows by a PVC in a 1:1 ratio.
- **Ventricular trigeminy PVC** PVC after two normal sinus beats.
- **Ventricular tachycardia** > than 100 bpm (or 120 bpm) wide QRS complex, a run of three or more PVCs. Sustain VT = run of VT >30 s.

Blocks

- **Sinus**

  Sinus block: Missed sinus P wave and QRS complex followed by resuming prior rhythm (if too prolong escape beat will occur).

  Sick Sinus Syndrome (SSS): Missing P waves and QRS complex without supra-ventricular escape beat mechanism (recurrent episodes of sinus block).

- **AV block** PR interval > 0.2 s.

  First degree: PR interval > 0.2 s (1 large EKG paper square) but constant intervals (P-P = P-P, P-R = P-R and R-R = R-R). QRS complex is preceded by a P wave.

  Second degree: Wenckebach (type I) prolongation of P-R intervals until a complete block in conduction with no QRS complex to follow. P-R ≠ P-R. These occur in a constant series of P:QRS ratios (4:3 or 5:4).

  Mobitz type II: P-P = P-P with R-R = R-R, with loss of QRS in a constant ratios of P:QRS (3:1, 2:1). Each cycle has P wave, not each cycle has QRS.

  Third degree: Complete block of atrial to ventricular depolarization. P-P = P-P and R-R = R-R. However, P-R ≠ P-R. No correlation between the P and the QRS complex. Rate of the ventricle will be dependent upon the location of the escape conduction (junctional focus → rate of 40–60 bpm, ventricular focus → 20–40 bpm).

- **LBBB** Wide QRS, left axis deviation, R-R′ in V_5 V_6 (R′ is left ventricular depolarization).
- **RBBB** Wide QRS, right axis deviation, R-R′ in V_1 V_2 (first R′ is right ventricular depolarization).

EKG Pathological Changes

- **Ischemia**   T wave symmetrical inversions of V2-V6. Subendocardial ischemia or ischemia due to stress test – flat ST depression (horizontal or downsloping).
- **Positive stress test criteria for ischemia on EKG**   > 1 mm depression of J point from baseline, persists at least 0.08 s (2 small boxes) after the J point for three consecutive beats at one or more leads (Fig. 8).
- **Acute injury/acute MI**   ST elevation: > 4 mm elevation of J point from baseline (Fig. 9).
- **Infarct/necrosis/scar**   Presence of Q wave – at least 1 mm wide OR 1/3 of the QRS amplitude (Fig. 10).

Fig. 8 > 1 mm depression of J point from baseline, persists at least 0.08 sec (2 small squares) after the J point for three consecutive beats in at least one or more leads

Fig. 9 > 4 mm elevation of J point from baseline

Fig. 10 Q wave – at least 1 mm wide OR 1/3 of the QRS amplitude

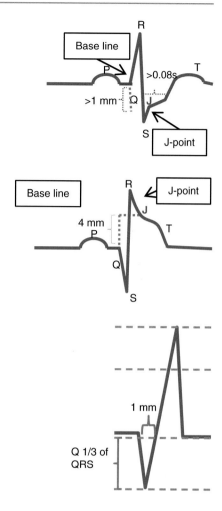

9.1   Flash Facts: EKG Tracing

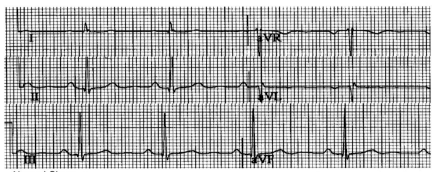

Normal Sinus

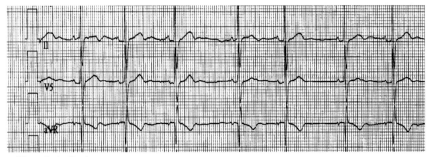

Sinus Arrhythmia

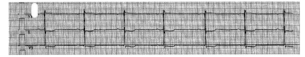

Sinus Bradycardia

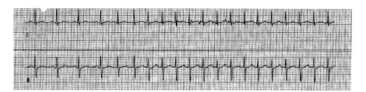

Paroxysmal Supraventricular Tachycardia

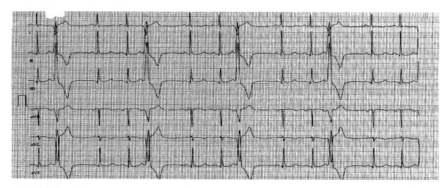

PVC-Trigeminy

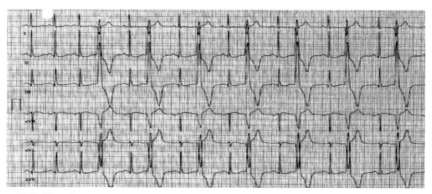

PVC-Bigeminy

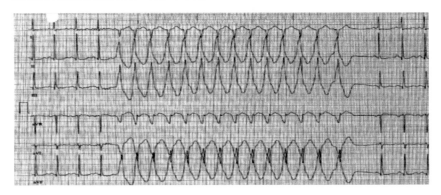

VT

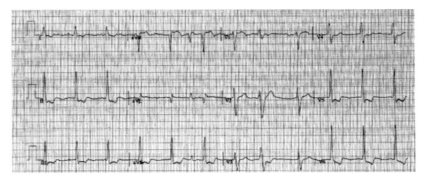

Inferolateral ischemia post regadenoson stress test.

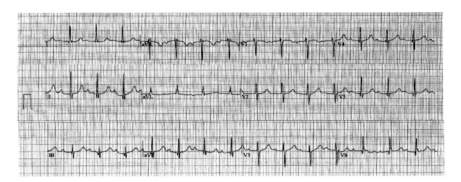

1st degree AV block

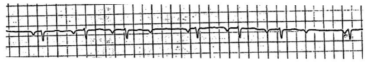

2nd degree AV block : Wenckeback (type I):

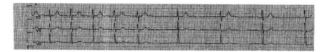

1st AV block progressed to 2nd degree block Mobitz Type II

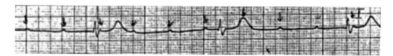

3st degree AV block

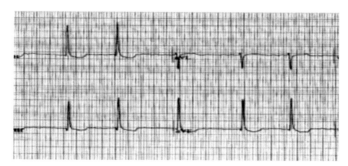

Digitalis effect

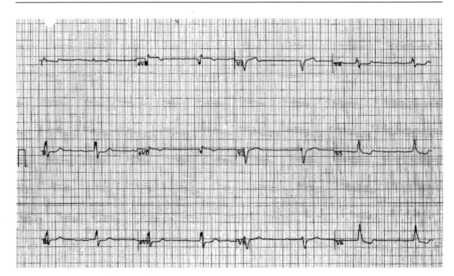

Left Bundle Branch block LBBB

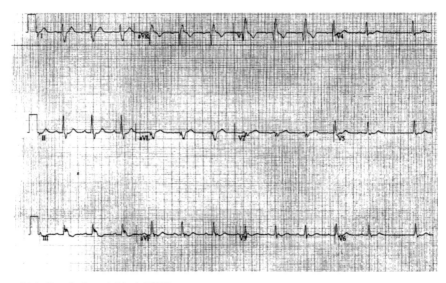

Right Bundle Branch block RBBB

Part 2: Clinical Nuclear Medicine – Head to Toe

Contents

© Springer International Publishing Switzerland 2017
B. Savir-Baruch, B.J. Barron, *RadTool Nuclear Medicine Flash Facts*,
DOI 10.1007/978-3-319-24636-9_2

1   Neurology

1.1   Cerebral Death Scan

Tracers   Tc-99m-HMPAO (Ceretec©), Tc-99m- ECD (Neurolite©), Tc-99m DTPA, Tc-99m Pertechnetate.

Tc-99m   Generator produced in the form of Tc-99m Pertechnetate (TcO$_4^{1-}$) from Mo-99. t_{phys} 6 h. *Emits* gamma 140 keV (89 %).

Tc-99m HMPAO/Tc-99m ECD   Lipophilic structure, crosses BBB, first-pass extraction of roughly 80 %. Not dependent on blood pressure, temperature, or cessation of phenobarbital.

Tc-99m DTPA/Tc-99m Pertechnetate   Flow agents – lipophobic: Do not cross BBB.

Mechanism *Tc-99m HMPAO/Tc-99m ECD*:   Blood pool → crosses BBB (lipophilic) → intracellular (cortical cell, via glutathione) → convert to hydrophilic complex → trapped → taken up by the mitochondria and the nucleus. Blue dye is used to stabilize the Tc-99m HMPAO molecule. It prevents the conversion of the Tc-99m HMPAO to a stereoisomeric form that rapidly washes out from the brain tissue. This may also be used as a quality control; blue color indicates the use of a brain agent. Useful when flow images were not obtained properly and carotids flow cannot be evaluated → no need to repeat exam if no brain uptake is noted by the end of the exam.
  Tc-99m DTPA and Tc-99m pertechnetate: IV bolus → flow to the internal carotid arteries → Circle of Willis to the anterior, middle, and posterior cerebellar arteries.

Dose   20 mCi. Negative study can be repeated in 6 h with 20 mCi of lipophobic tracers or *x*2 the initial dose of lipophilic tracer.

Protocol: IV bolus → angiographic phase (flow images) 1 s/frame for 1 min. Blood pool phase: Anterior and lateral images until 500 K counts for 10–20 min with lipophilic tracer +/− SPECT. Or immediate and 10 min delay images with lipophobic tracers.

Target Organ *Bladder:* Tc-99m ECD, Tc-99m DTPA, Tc-99m pertechnetate. *Lacrimal gland:* Tc-99m-HMPAO.

Negative Scan *Lipophilic tracer:* Uptake within brain parenchyma. *Lipophobic tracer* angiographic phase: Visualization of "trident sign" (anterior and middle cerebellar arteries); blood pool phase: Visualization of venous sinuses.

Positive Scan (brain death):
  Lipophilic tracer: No uptake within brain parenchyma. Increase nasal uptake.
  Lipophobic tracer: angiographic phase: No "trident sign" with an "empty bulb" appearance (only scalp perfusion from external carotid with no brain perfusion). Blood pool phase: May or may not see venous sinuses.

False Positive Absence of angiography phase with lipophobic tracers. Use tracer that does not cross BBB (obtaining flow phase is important even with lipophilic tracers).

False Negative Scalp perfusion on lateral images mimics brain perfusion – apply tourniquet (absolute contraindication in small children).

Poor Prognostic Signs *Tc-99m DTPA/Tc-99m pertechnetate*: No flow noted on angiography phase, with a sagittal sinus sign on delay phase images (may also be false negative). *Tc-99m HMPAO/Tc-99m ECD* "Helmet sign" – no perfusion to brain stem and cerebellum. Persistent cerebral perfusion.

Distribution and Clearance

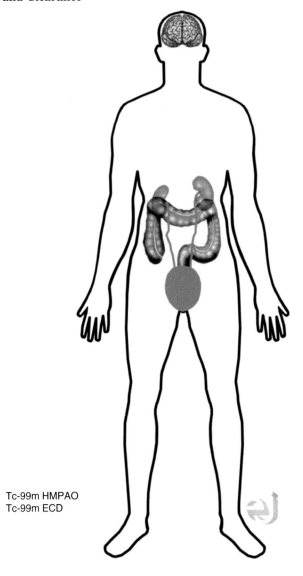

Tc-99m HMPAO
Tc-99m ECD

Distribution Trapped in the brain (intracellular, trapped); muscle and soft tissue (not trapped).
Clearance By decay in the brain (trapped). Kidneys and hepatobiliary (not trapped).

Distribution and Clearance: Brain-Specific Agents

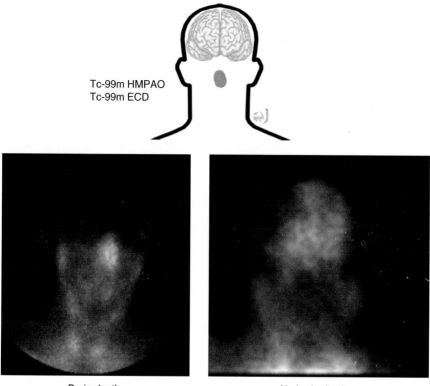

Tc-99m HMPAO
Tc-99m ECD

Brain death   No brain death

Distribution and Clearance: Brain Nonspecific Agents

Patient progressed from a negative to a positive brain perfusion scan. Fig. A – flow study demonstrates visualization of "trident sign" on arterial flow phase. Ten-minute delay image demonstrates appearance of a sagittal sinus. Fig. B – on a repeated study 3 days later, a complete loss of brain perfusion is noted on flow images, as well as loss of sagittal sinus uptake on 10 min delay images.

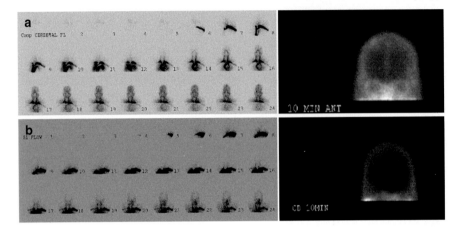

1.2 Brain Scan: Dementia and Epilepsy

Indications *Cerebral perfusion* and metabolism (dementia, epilepsy, and brain death).

Tc-99m Generator produced in the form of Tc-99m pertechnetate (TcO_4^{1-}) from Mo-99. t_{phys} 6 h, *emits* gamma 140 keV.

Tc-99m HMPAO/Tc-99m ECD Lipophilic structure, crosses BBB, first-pass extraction of roughly 80 %.

Mechanism *Cerebral flow:* Blood pool → crosses BBB (lipophilic) → intracellular (cortical cell, via glutathione) → convert to hydrophilic complex → trapped → taken by the mitochondria and the nucleus. *Tc-99m ECD has a longer shelf life, which permits longer delay in administration while waiting on ictal activity to be demonstrated on EEG.*

F-18 Cyclotron produced. t_{phys} 109.8 min. *Decay:* Positron emission; gamma ray energy = 511 keV. Decays to O-18.

F-18 FDG (*fluorodeoxyglucose*) is a glucose metabolism agent.

Mechanism FDG-6P → trapped in cell (missing 2'OH group needed for metabolism). After full decay from F-18 to O-18 (heavy oxygen), it will combine with H^+ ion to create 2'OH group that will be metabolized in glycolysis.

Brain scan: Will demonstrate changes in cerebral glucose metabolism associated with foci of epileptic seizures/tumors/dementia.

Dose *Cerebral flow:* 20 mCi. *Metabolism* 10–15 mCi.

Protocol

Tc-99m HMPAO/Tc-99m ECD: IV (Ceretec©) or Tc-99m ECD (Neurolite©) → 15 min-2 h postinjection SPECT as close as possible to the head. *Ictal*: done with SPECT under EEG monitoring → inject at the time of seizure. (FDG t_{phys} is too short and preparation is needed).

FDG: Fasting for 4 h (brain) → IV FDG → "cooking" time for 45 min to 1 h. → CT (attenuation correction) and PET images.

Critical Organ *Tc-99m HMPAO* lacrimal glands. *F-18 FDG* Bladder.

Abnormal Brain Distribution Patterns

- *Alzheimer's disease*: Decreased uptake within the temporal parietal cortex with sparing of the frontal lobe, basal ganglia, thalamus, and cerebellum. Posterior cingulate gyrus is often first to go.
- *Lewy Body dementia*: Decreased uptake within the temporal parietal cortex and occipital lobes with sparing of the cerebellum, basal ganglia, and thalamus.
- *Frontotemporal dementias*: Decreased uptake within the frontal lobe, sparing posterior parietal regions.
- *Vascular dementia*: Diffuse decreased uptake within multiple locations. Can be wedge shaped.
- *Epilepsy:* Ictal: Asymmetrically increased perfusion to the epileptic focus (FDG PET is not used in this phase). Interictal (less sensitive phase than ictal): Asymmetrically decreased perfusion to the epileptic focus (with SPECT) or hypometabolism within the epileptic focus (with FDG PET). FDG PET is slightly more sensitive than SPECT.

Distribution: *Tc-99m HMPAO/Tc-99m ECD*: Trapped in the brain (intracellular, trapped); muscle and soft tissue (not trapped). F-18 *FDG*: Brain >> kidneys, ureters, and bladder >> liver, variable: heart, GI, salivary glands, uterus, ovaries, and testes.

Clearance *Tc-99m HMPAO:* By decay in the brain (trapped). Kidneys and hepato-biliary (not trapped). F-18 *FDG*: kidneys, ureters, and bladder.

Distribution and Clearance

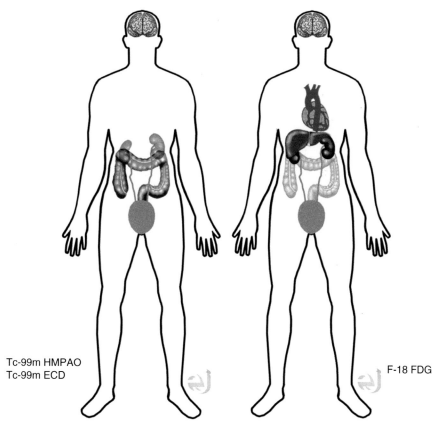

Tc-99m HMPAO
Tc-99m ECD

F-18 FDG

Distribution *Tc-99m HMPAO* Trapped in the brain (intracellular, trapped); muscle and soft tissue (not trapped). *F-18 FDG*: Brain >> kidneys, ureters, and bladder >> liver. Variable: Heart, GI, salivary glands, uterus, spleen, ovaries, and testes.
Clearance *Tc-99m HMPAO* By decay in the brain (trapped). Kidneys and hepatobiliary (not trapped). *F-18 FDG*: kidneys, ureters, and bladder.

Distribution Patterns: Normal

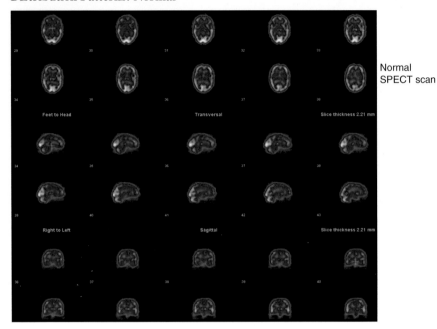

Normal
SPECT scan

Abnormal Distribution

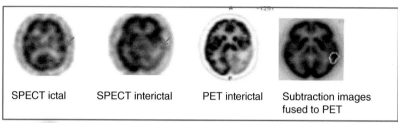

| SPECT ictal | SPECT interictal | PET interictal | Subtraction images fused to PET |

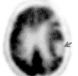

PET. MCA
infarct

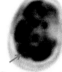

Crossed cerebellar
diaschisis

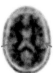

Lewy body disease

Alzheimer's disease

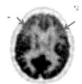

Frontotemporal dementia

1.3   I-123 Ioflupane (DaTscan)

Indication Evaluation of patients presenting with dopaminergic symptoms to differentiate parkinsonian syndromes from essential tremors.

I-123 Cyclotron-produced t_{phys} 13.3 h. *Emits* gamma photons 159 KeV.

Additional I-123 Uses Thyroid uptake and scan, whole-body scan for thyroid cancer and I-123 MIBG scan.

Ioflupane Dopamine Transporter (DaT) visualization agent. Cocaine analog. Phenyltropane compound.

Mechanism Isoflurane has high binding affinity (reversible) for presynaptic dopamine transporters (DaT) in the striatal region of the brain. Loss of DaT significantly correlates with loss of nigrostriatal neurons in Parkinson disease.

Side Effects Headache, vertigo, increased appetite, and tactile hallucinations. Accepted medical use with strict inventory. Classified as DEA Schedule II controlled substance due to abuse and dependence potential.

Protocol *Preparation*: 1 h prior – 5 drops of thyroid-blocking agent Lugol's Solution orally. May also use SSKI Solution.

Dose 3 to 5 mCi IV.

Image 3–6 h postinjection, brain SPECT images (approx 30 min).

Interpretation *Normal:* Human striatal anatomy, comma shape. *Abnormal:* Right or left asymmetry within the putamen or caudate nucleus structures, or bilateral decrease/change of normal comma shape.

Critical Organ Bladder.

Distribution Consistent with human striatal anatomy (peak uptake 3–6 h with 30 %).

Clearance By 48 h postinjection, 60 % will be excreted via urine, 14 % GI.

Distribution and Clearance

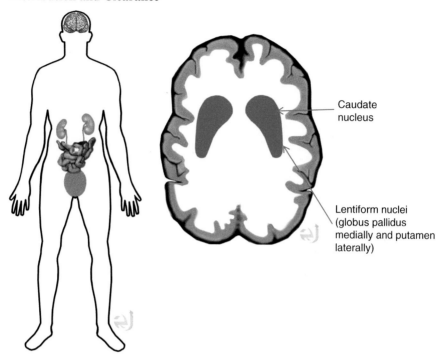

Caudate nucleus

Lentiform nuclei (globus pallidus medially and putamen laterally)

Distribution Consistent with human striatal anatomy (peak uptake 3–6 h with 30 %).

Clearance By 48 h postinjection, 60 % will be excreted via urine, 14 % GI.

Distribution Patterns: Normal

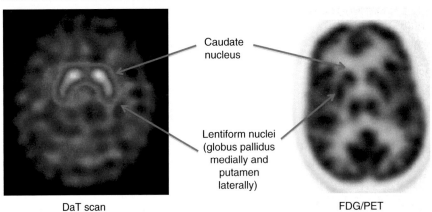

Caudate
nucleus

Lentiform nuclei
(globus pallidus
medially and
putamen
laterally)

DaT scan   FDG/PET

Distribution Patterns: Abnormal

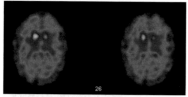

Persistent caudate nucleus, with some loss of putamen, left worse than right

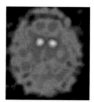

Persistent caudate nucleus, with complete loss of putamen

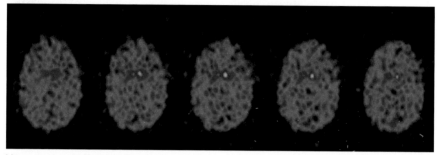

Young man with Ecstasy damage

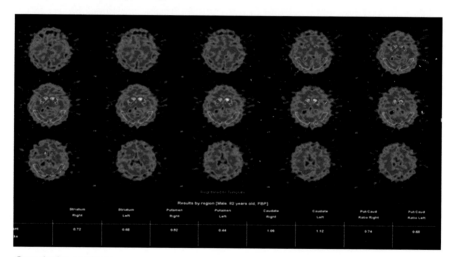

Results by region [Male 82 years old, FBP]

Striatum Right	Striatum Left	Putamen Right	Putamen Left	Caudate Right	Caudate Left	Put Caud Ratio Right	Put Caud Ratio Left
0.72	0.68	0.52	0.44	1.06	1.12	0.74	0.68

Quantitation analysis

Semi-quantitative Ratios of region interest (ROI) of highly binding DaT structures (striatum) with ROI of low binding DaT structures such as the occipital lobe. Striatal binding ratio = [mean counts of striatal ROI - mean counts of occipital ROI]/mean counts of occipital ROI.

1.4   Indium-111 DTPA Cisternography

Indications Cerebral spine fluid (CSF) circulation: (1) Hydrocephalus, (2) CSF leak, (3) ventriculoperitoneal (VP) or ventriculoatrial (VA) shunt patency.

Indium-111 Cyclotron produced from cadmium (Cd-112) target. t_{phys} 2.83 days (67 h). *Decays*: Electron Capture (EC). *Emits*: gamma 173 keV (89 %) and 247 keV (94 %).

DTPA (Diethylenetriaminepentaacetic Acid) A polyaminopolycarboxylic acid *chelator*, similar to ethylenediaminetetraacetic acid (EDTA) derivatives.

Mechanism Intrathecal injection of the radiopharmaceutical; will slowly be absorbed in the subarachnoid space which allows tracking of CSF flow dynamics.

Dose 0.5 mCi in 10 % dextrose. Lumbar puncture (LP) and intrathecal injection of the radiotracer.

Hydrocephalus *Concept of normal CSF production and flow* CSF will be produced predominantly by the choroid plexus of the lateral, 3rd, and 4th ventricles which will determine the dynamics of normal flow. *At any time point, there will be no reverse flow toward the lateral ventricles in a normal individual. Normal CSF flow*: Lateral ventricle (*CSF production*) → 3rd vertical via the foramen of Monro (*CSF production*) → flow via the cerebral aqueduct of Sylvius → 4th vertical (*CSF production*) → spinal cord subarachnoid via the foramen of Magendie and two Luschka foramina → basal cisterns → subarachnoid over the convexities.

Protocol Image at 1 h postinjection, 3–4 and 24 h postinjection images of the head and spine in the vertex, anterior, posterior, and lateral projections. 48 h images as needed.
   Normal flow following intrathecal injection: Basal cistern activity shows in 4 h images → tracer over the entire convexities in 24 h.
   Abnormal flow: Brain atrophy due to age: Delay migration of the tracer over the convexities – no lateral ventricles are seen. Communicating hydrocephalus (normal pressure hydrocephalus) → visualization of the lateral ventricles without migration of tracer over the convexities.

Nasal CSF Leak *Protocol*: Intrathecal injection followed by insertion (usually by ENT) of 6 nasal meatus pledgets labeled as superior, middle, and inferior nasal meatus, bilaterally (1–6). Image protocol may vary per location of the radiotracer with time – image at 1 h, followed by 4 and 24 h as needed. Once full migration of the tracer is seen → remove the pledgets → place each in a test tube → measure and record counts of each pledget with a well counter. Draw 10 ml of blood, measure, and record counts. *Interpretation*: Pledgets counts/plasma counts > 2.5–3 are abnormal. Use pledget labels for accurate localization. *Ear CSF leak*: Look for asymmetry in the images.

Shunt Patency *Protocol*: Inject tracer into a scalp shunt reservoir or via LP. Images at 10 min, 1 h, 6 h and 24 h to confirm migration of the tracer into the peritoneum with ventriculoperitoneal shunts or intravascular with ventriculoatrial shunt.

Critical Organ Spinal cord.

Pitfalls: In-111, DTPA is used in adults with the advantage of longer half-life and the need of delay images. However, it is not recommended in pediatric population due to high radiation. Tc-99m DTPA may be used instead.

Distribution CSF flow dynamics.

Clearance Absorption of labeled CSF into the blood by the arachnoid villi and by the cerebral and spinal leptomeninges in a lesser extent. Within the first 24 h, approximately 65 % of the dose will be excreted by the kidneys and 85 % at 72 h postinjection.

Distribution and Clearance

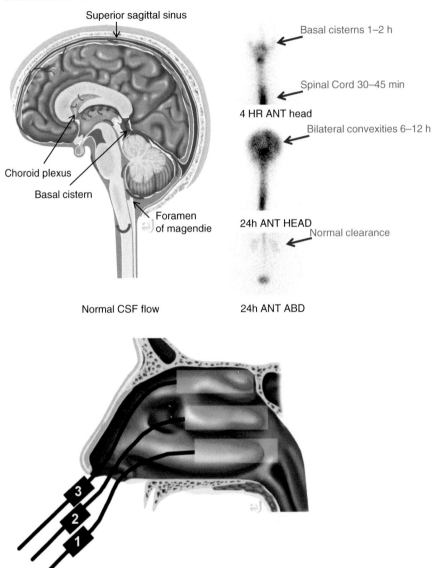

Superior sagittal sinus

Choroid plexus

Basal cistern

Foramen of magendie

Normal CSF flow

Basal cisterns 1–2 h

Spinal Cord 30–45 min

4 HR ANT head

Bilateral convexities 6–12 h

24h ANT HEAD
Normal clearance

24h ANT ABD

Normal placement nasal meatus labeled pledgets

Distribution CSF flow dynamics.

Clearance Absorption of labeled CSF into the blood by the arachnoid villi and by the cerebral and spinal leptomeninges in a lesser extent. Within the first 24 h, approximately 65 % of the dose will be excreted by the kidneys and 85 % in 72 h postinjection.

Normal Distribution and Clearance

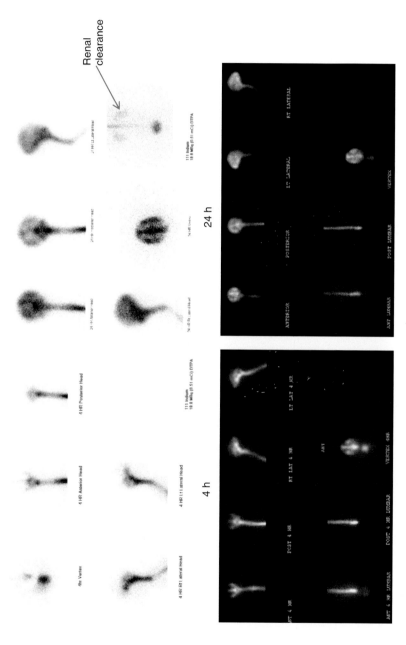

Abnormal Distribution

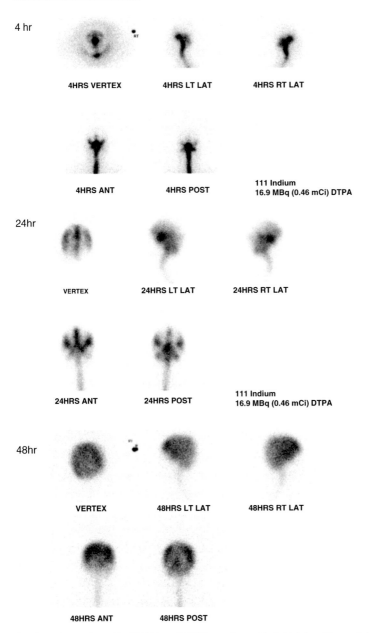

4 hr

4HRS VERTEX   4HRS LT LAT   4HRS RT LAT

4HRS ANT   4HRS POST

111 Indium
16.9 MBq (0.46 mCi) DTPA

24hr

VERTEX   24HRS LT LAT   24HRS RT LAT

24HRS ANT   24HRS POST

111 Indium
16.9 MBq (0.46 mCi) DTPA

48hr

VERTEX   48HRS LT LAT   48HRS RT LAT

48HRS ANT   48HRS POST

Elderly patient evaluated for NPH-Normal CSF flow pattern with slight delay of tracer distribution within the convexities. Normal variant to age due to atrophy.

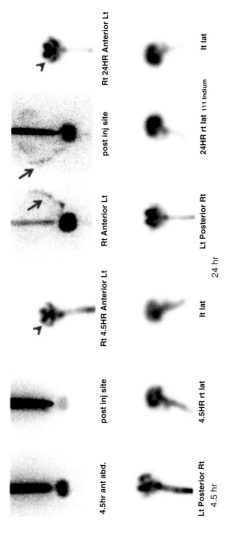

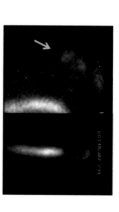

Patent with NPH- After placing VP shunt. Persistent tracer within the lateral ventricles (*arrow head*). At 24 hr, there is failure of tracer to migration over the convexities, characteristic of NPH. VP shunt is patent (*arrow*).

Patent VP shunt- In-111 DTPA in the peritoneal cavity 24 hr. post LP injection

2   Eyes

2.1   Dacryoscintigraphy

The technique of Dacryoscintigraphy (DS) has not been standardized, with several protocols existing in the literature.

Tracers Tc-99m pertechnetate or Tc-99m sulfur colloid.

Purpose Evaluation of lacrimal drainage patency (epiphora – overflow of tears onto the face).

Tc-99m Generator produced in the form of Tc-99m pertechnetate (TcO$_4^{1-}$) (+7 valence) from Mo-99. t_{phys} 6 h *Emits* gamma 140 keV (89 %).

Dose 0.1 mCi.

Mechanism Direct application of tracer to the eye will demonstrate the normal pattern of tear drainage. (Optimal with special dispenser).

Protocol Tracer instilled in the inferior fornix simultaneously or near simultaneously via a micropipette, preferably, or a syringe. The volume per eye ranges from 10 to 25 μl (with smaller volumes, it is less likely to cause overflow of tracer onto the cheek).

Image Patient seated/supine with their cornea less than 2 cm from the collimator (LEAP or LEHR typically, pinholes have been used). Dynamic images (1 min frames for 10–15 min or 10–30 s frames for several min). Static images up to 45 min after instillation.

Target Organ Lens.

Interpretation Pre-lacrimal sac (pre-sac) delay → tracer fails to reach the sac by 2–3 min, pre-ductal delay → no sac emptying is seen by 3–5 min, and ductal delay if tracer has not entered the nose by 6 min. Delay to drainage defined as mild (6–15 min), moderate (16–30), and severe (31–45).

Distribution Patterns: Normal

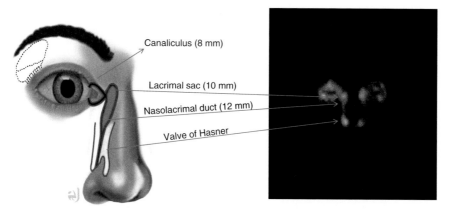

Canaliculus (8 mm)

Lacrimal sac (10 mm)

Nasolacrimal duct (12 mm)

Valve of Hasner

Distribution Patterns: Normal

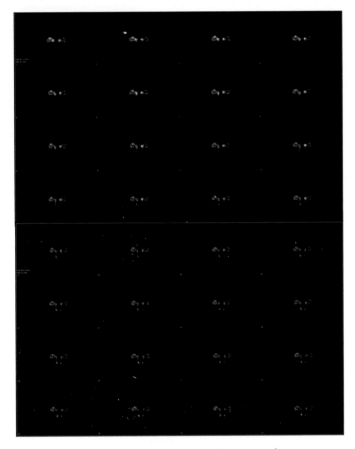

Dynamic images of the first 8 min, 15 sec per frame
demonstrate normal movement of the tracer into the
lacrimal sac and normal drainage through the
nasolacrimal ducts bilaterally

Distribution Patterns: Abnormal

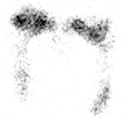

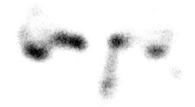

Bilateral epiphora: No tracer movement into the lacrimal sac (pre-sac delay) bilaterally on a 20 min static image. Tear overflow onto the cheeks is also seen

Persistence of tracer in the right lacrimal sac (post-sac delay) on a 20 min static image. No movement into the nasolacrimal duct. Patent left system

3 Neck

3.1 Thyroid Uptake and Scan

Indication Hyperthyroidism, thyroid nodule, neonatal hypothyroidism.

I-123 (Oral) Cyclotron-produced t_{phys} 13.3 h *Emits* gamma photons 159 keV.

Tc-99m Pertechnetate (for IV Administration) Mo-99 generator-produced t_{phys} 6 h. *Emits* gamma 140 keV.

Mechanism

I-123 Na Iodide Rapid GI absorption of iodine in the extracellular fluid → active uptake in the thyroid follicles by Na/I symporter → protein-bound iodine (organification). Chemical form T_3 and T_4. All drugs which affect the thyroid hormone synthesis pathway (Synthroid, PTU, Tapazole, Armour Thyroid) will affect iodine uptake (highly regulated by TSH). Additional uptake (non-protein-bound uptake mechanism) by salivary glands, stomach cells (no trapping), and hepatocytes (thyroglobulin metabolism).

Tc-99m Pertechnetate will be transported via the I/Na Symporter channel to the thyroid follicles without organification → No trapping; will wash out with time.

Dose *Adult: I-123 NaI* (0.1–0.3 mCi). *Tc-99m pertechnetate* (2–10 mCi). *Children: I-123 NaI* (0.1–0.2 mCi). *Tc-99m pertechnetate* 1–5 mCi.

Protocol *preparation:* stop Tapazole, Methimazole, and PTU for 3 days; no iodinated contrast study in the last 6 weeks. Stop Amiodarone 3–6 m prior to treatment.
    Image: At 24 h with I-123 NaI or at 2 h with Tc-99m pertechnetate. Using a LEHR collimator, acquire anterior images followed by pinhole images in ANT, RAO, and LAO projections.

Interpretation

1. I-123 NaI
   - Hyperthyroidism: Thyroid uptake at 24 h (uptake at 4 h is optional). Normal range is 10–35 % at 24 h and 6–18 % at 4 h .
     Assumption: The capsule is counted at T_0 and the thyroid is counted at T_{24}. Formula for I-123: Use a 24 h decay factor = 0.2863.

$$\% \text{Uptake at T}_{24} = \frac{\left\{\left[\text{Neck counts}(\text{CPM}) - \text{Thigh counts}(\text{CPM})\right] \times 100\ \%\right\}}{\left\{0.2863\left[\text{Capsule counts}(\text{CPM}) - \text{Room background counts}(\text{CPM})\right]\right\}}$$

2. Tc-99m pertechnetate and I-123 NaI
   - Evaluation of thyroid nodules: Decreased uptake (cold nodule) associated with 15–20 % chance of malignancy → biopsy.
3. Tc-99m pertechnetate
   - Evaluation of thyroid agenesis/lingual thyroid in neonates with hypothyroidism: If uptake is noted in the thyroid bed → evaluate for organification failure with I-123 scan.
   - Evaluation of thyroid nodules: If increased uptake is noted on TcO_4^{1-} (hot nodule) → perform I-123 scan → if no uptake → discordant nodule (positive on Tc-99m and negative on I-123 scans) → biopsy (15–20 % chance of malignancy).

Critical Organ Thyroid.

Concept Once TSH < 0.1 mIU/L → no uptake will be demonstrated in a normal regulated thyroid cell due to negative pituitary-thyroid feedback.
TSH < 0.1 mIU/L with homogenous uptake in thyroid gland: Graves – if uptake is less than 30 % → look for history of recent large iodine uptake such as multivitamins or contrast CT.
TSH < 0.1 mIU/L with heterogamous uptake in thyroid gland: Multinodular goiter.
TSH < 0.1 mIU/L with one "hot" nodule and no uptake in the surrounded thyroid tissue: Toxic nodule.
TSH < 0.1 mIU/L with no uptake in the thyroid tissue: Subacute thyroiditis or factitious thyroiditis.

Distribution Iodine-containing tissue (thyroid tissue, salivary gland, and stomach) + GI lumen (oral admin), 7 days post-scan – liver uptake due to thyroid hormone metabolism.

Clearance Renal, metabolized in the liver.

Suggested Reading
- Society of Nuclear Medicine Procedure Guideline for Therapy of Thyroid Disease with Iodine-131 (Sodium Iodide) 3.0

Distribution and Clearance

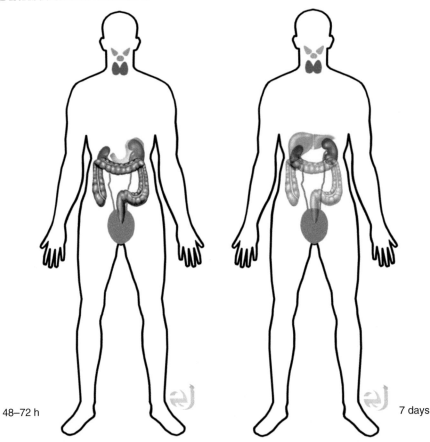

48–72 h

7 days

Distribution Iodine-containing tissue (thyroid tissue, salivary gland, and stomach) + GI lumen (oral admin).

Clearance By kidneys, metabolized in the liver.

Normal Distribution

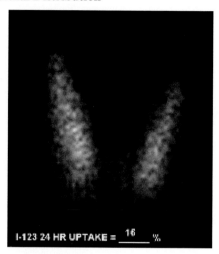

I-123 24 HR UPTAKE = _16_ %

Normal thyroid uptake scan
with 24hr uptake of <30 %

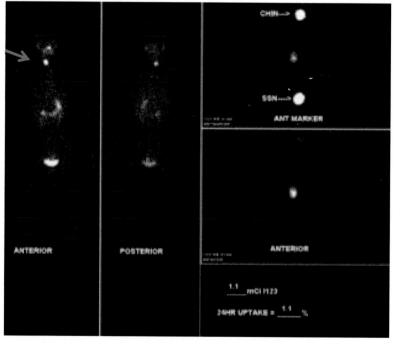

Whole body iodine scan in a patient with thyroid cancer after total thyroidectomy.
Post-surgical expected minimal thyroid bed residual uptake (arrow).

Distribution Iodine-avid tissue (thyroid tissue, salivary gland, and stomach)+GI lumen (oral admin).
Clearance By kidneys, metabolized in the liver.

Abnormal Distribution

Low TSH. High T_3/T_4

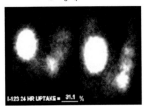

Multinodular goiter:
multiple hot nodules

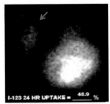

Toxic node: single large nodule with
suppressed adjacent thyroid tissue.

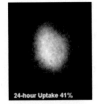

Graves with agenesis
of single thyroid lobe

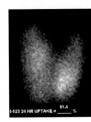

Graves'disease:
homogenous high thyroid uptake.

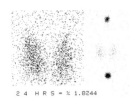

Subacute thyroiditis or factitious thyroiditis: Low
to no thyroid uptake.

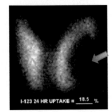

*Cold nodule

- Paradox: cold nodule is not completely "cold"and therefore ablation with I131 is the first line choice after resection. Thyroid cancer cells will take the iodine but to a lesser degree than that of a benign hyperfunctional tissue.

3.2 Tc-99m Sestamibi (MIBI): Parathyroid Scan

Indications Parathyroid adenoma, elevated PTH with hypercalcemia.

Other Uses Cardiac stress scan, breast cancer.

Tc-99m Generator produced in the form of Tc-99m pertechnetate (TcO_4^{1-}) (+7 valence) from Mo-99. t_{phys} 6 h *emits* gamma 140 keV (89 %).

Mechanism
- *Lipophilic structure*: Passive diffuse to the cell → uptake by mitochondria due to membrane electric potential → retention due to electrostatic interactions → trapped within the mitochondria.
- *Oxyphil cells:* Secreting cell → higher mitochondria concentration → higher tracer retention. Parathyroid adenoma expression of oxyphil secretion cells is higher than normal thyroid gland.
- Washout by Pgp (P glycoprotein). Tumor cell [Pgp] expression is related to tumor drug resistance (used in breast CA).

Protocol IV injection of Tc-99m sestamibi. Early images – anterior static images at 10–15 min of neck and upper chest → delay anterior static images at 1–2 h with or without SPECT/CT, institution dependent.

Dose 20 mCi.

Image Interpretation
- *Normal*: Early images – homogeneous tracer uptake within the thyroid. Delay: Thyroid tracer washout.
- *Abnormal*: Early images – homogeneous/heterogeneous uptake within the thyroid gland. Delayed image: Thyroid tracer washout with persistent uptake within a parathyroid gland. No retention of tracer in delay images may indicate early washout from a clear cell parathyroid adenoma.

Ectopic Parathyroid Adenoma Intrathyroidal, along the thyroid bed toward the thymic bed, thymus, carotid artery sheath, mediastinum, along the esophagus, and retropharyngeal space.
  Hyperplasia: Visualization of all four glands.

Distribution *Early 30 min:* Thyroid salivary gland, heart >>> liver, kidney.
Late >60 min: Biliary tract, GI, kidney, bladder > liver, heart >> thyroid, salivary gland.

Clearance Bile to GI and kidney.

Suggested Reading
- GOMES, Elaine Maria Santos et al (2007) Ectopic and extranumerary parathyroid gland location in patients with hyperparathyroidism secondary to end-stage renal disease. Acta Cir Bras. [online]. 22(2)

Distribution and Clearance

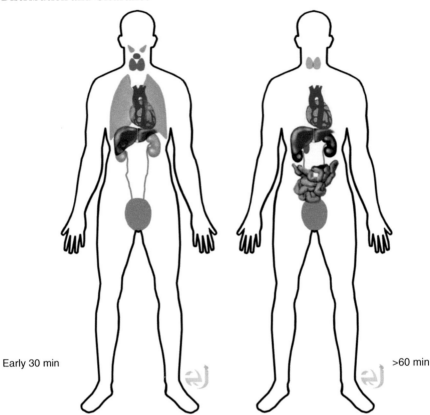

Early 30 min   >60 min

Distribution
Early 30 min: Thyroid salivary gland, heart >>> liver, kidney.

Late >60 min: Biliary tract, GI, kidney, bladder > liver, heart >> thyroid, salivary gland.

Clearance Bile to GI and kidney.

Normal Distribution

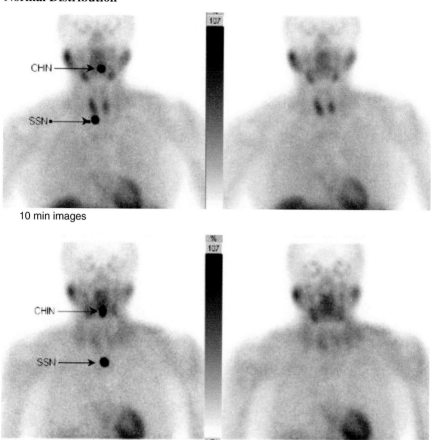

10 min images

2 h. delayed images - Near complete tracer washout from the thyroid gland.

CHN and SSN: Sealed markers; chin and sternal notch.

Abnormal Distribution

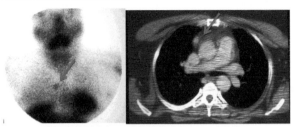

Ectopic Parathyroid Adenoma

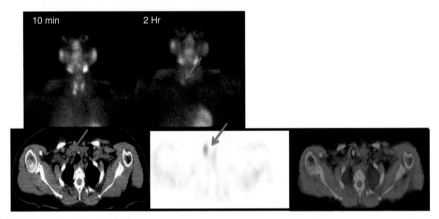

Right lower Parathyroid Adenoma

4   Lungs

4.1   V/Q Scan: Ventilation

Indications Acute pulmonary embolism. Also, chronic pulmonary embolism due to pulmonary hypertension.

Ventilation Imaging Obtained usually before perfusion. *Xe-133/Tc-99m* MAA: Prevents down scatter energy of higher energy (140–80 keV). *Tc/Tc exam*: lower dose ratio for ventilation (1 mCi Tc-99m DTPA vs. 3–6 mCi of Tc-99m MAA).

Xenon 133 Gas (Xe 133) Nuclear Reactor (Fission of U-235), Lipophilic. t_{phys} 5 days, t_{biol} 30 s. *Decays:* Beta minus. *Emits:* 81 keV gamma *dose* 10–30 mCi. *Target Organ:* Lungs. Operation requires a negative-pressure room.

Image Protocol Gas is inhaled via a closed system using face mask/mouthpiece:
1. *Single-breath phase*: Patient breathes Xe-133. Patient takes one deep breath and holds his/her breath.
2. *Equilibrium phase*: Patient breathes mixed air and Xe-133.
3. *Washout phase*: Breathes only air. Exhaled Xe-133 delivered to activated charcoal trapping system.

Imaging
- *Method 1 – Xenon phase performed prior to perfusion*: Three anterior/posterior spot images are obtained for each phase (total of nine images). Advantage – no down scatter of higher energy. Disadvantage: All patients required ventilation in the anterior posterior projection.
- *Method 2 – Xenon phase performed after perfusion*: Will be performed only if perfusion images are suspicious for pulmonary embolism. Xenon images will be obtained in the required projection with three images for each phase (total of nine images). Advantage – patients required ventilation in the clinically indicated projection (after review of perfusion images). Patients may not be ventilated at all. Disadvantage: Down scatter of higher energy is present.

Normal Distribution
- Homogenous tracer distribution and washout (no defects or trapping).

Abnormal Distribution
- *Single-breath and equilibrium phases*: Normal/slow/no tracer filling.
- *Washout phase*: Tracer trapping/no filling.

Tc-99m-DTPA

Tc-99m: Generator produced in the form of Tc-99m pertechnetate (TcO_4^{1-}) (+7 valence) from Mo-99. t_{phys} 6 h. **Emits** gamma 140 keV (89 %).

DTPA Aerosol Particle Size 0.1–0.5 µm. Aerosolized by nebulizer.

Mechanism Aerosols precipitate in airway mucosa → crossing the airway membrane → entering the circulation → cleared by the kidney.

t_{biol} is 60–100 min in healthy people and ~25 min in smokers.

Target Organ Bladder.

Dose 30–45 mCi liquid is aerosolized by nebulizer to administer a total dose equal to 1–2 mCi.

Imaging Protocol After breathing the aerosols via mouthpiece with nose clip for several min, images can be obtain. (A) multi planar views: ANT/POS, RL/LL, RAO/LPO, LAO/LPO. Or (B) SPECT.

Distribution

Normal: Homogenous tracer distribution (no defects or clumping).

Abnormal: Heterogeneous distribution, cold defects, clumping.

Technetium-99m Technegas Tc-99m-labeled solid graphite particles (0.005–0.2 µm) in argon carrier gas (gas and particle properties).

Preparation *Technegas generator:* In a crucible, Tc-99m-pertechnetate is heated to high temperatures in the presence of argon gas to create labeled Tc-99m-carbon particle encapsulated within a layer of graphite carbon.

Mechanism Particles carried to the alveoli by the argon gas and adhere to alveoli mucosa.

Benefits No central clumping and advantage of performing multiview planar images or SPECT.

Target Organ Lung

Dose 20 mCi of Tc-99m is inserted to the Technegas generator to administer a total dose of 1 mCi.

Protocol Radiopharmaceutical delivered to the patient via Technegas generator contains Tc-99m-labeled graphite particle in argon gas. *(1)* Supine position, *(2)* nose clip + mouthpiece on, *(3)* deep breathe and hold for 3 s, *(4)* exhale, *(5)* repeat two to three times.

Images (A) Multiview planar images: Ant/Pos, RL/LL, RAO/LPO, LAO/LPO. Or (B) SPECT.

Distribution

Normal: Homogenous tracer distribution (no defects or clumping).

Abnormal: Heterogeneous distribution, cold defects.

Extrapulmonary Distribution *Xenon*: Liver uptake – Fatty liver, fatty marrow. *Aerosols*: Oral cavity, esophagus. Stomach – swallow of particles.

4.2   V/Q Scan: Perfusion

Indication Acute pulmonary embolism. *Other indications:* Chronic pulmonary embolism due to pulmonary hypertension.

Perfusion Study Obtain after ventilation. *Xe-133/Tc-99m MAA* – Prevents down scatter of higher energy (140–80 keV). *Tc/Tc exam* – lower dose ratio for ventilation (1 mCi Tc-99m DTPA vs. 3–6 mCi of Tc-99m MAA).

Tc-99m Generator produced in the form of Tc 99m pertechnetate (TcO_4^{1-}) (+7 valence) from Mo-99. t_{phys} 6 h. *Emits* gamma 140 keV (89 %).

Macroaggregated Albumin (MAA) Particles Size: 90 % between 10–90 μm and 0 % > 150 μm; actual range: 20–40 μm. Particles in a size of 1 to ~7 μm are taken up by the reticuloendothelial system (RES). *MAA Kit* – contains four to eight million MAA particles and stannous ion (to reduce TcO_4^{1-} oxidation state from +7 to +4). Each vial should be reconstituted with up to 100 mCi of Tc-99m pertechnetate.

Tc-99m-MAA: Mechanism of Localization (known as "capillary blockade"): t_{biol} 2–3 h. MAA particles are larger than the capillaries. Hence, once injected via the venous system, they will be trapped within the pulmonary alveolar capillary bed.

Study Protocol
   Dose: *Healthy adult*: 1–6 mCi, 200–700K MAA particles; ideal number: 350 K with a minimum of 200 K particles. *Pulmonary hypertension patient*: maximum of 150 K particles. *Dose modification* 1–3 mCi pregnant (preferred perfusion only with 150 K MAA); known right to left shunt and chronic pulmonary hypertension (1–3 mCi, 150 K particles MAA V/Q). *Pediatric* 25–50 μCi/kg. *Newborn* 200–500 μCi.
   Imaging (A) Multiview planar images: ANT/POS, RL/LL, RAO/LPO, LAO/LPO. (B) Lung SPECT.

Critical Organ Lung.

Distribution Pulmonary alveolar capillary bed.
   Abnormal distribution (*no PE*) (**A**) right-to-left cardiac shunt: lung, brain, kidneys (**B**). SVC occlusion: lung, hepatic caudate lobe. (**C**) Atrial-venous collaterals: lung, kidneys, no brain. (**D**) Edge scalloping: microemboli due to fat, sepsis, air, tumor, amniotic fluid.

Clearance MAA particles are fragile and will undergo degradation to be phagocytized in the RES (reticuloendothelial system in the liver and spleen).

4.3   V/Q Interpretation

Pre-test Risk Probability of PE

Well's criteria[a]	
DVT (diagnosis, clinical signs, symptoms)	3 points
PE is highly suspected	3 points
HR is > 100 bpm	1.5 points
Immobilization > 3 days ar Surgery in the past 4 weeks	1.5 points
Prior history of DVT or PE	1.5 points
Hemoptysis	1 point
Malignancy undergoing treatment in the past 6 m	1 point

DVT Deep vain thrombosis, *PE* Pulmonary embolism, *HR* Heart rate

Score
Well's criteria

- 1–2.0 points: Low risk with 15 % probability of PE
- 2.5–6.0 points: Moderate risk with 29 % probability of PE
- 6.5–12.5 points: High Risk with 56 % probability of PE
- OR:
- ≤4 PE unlikely
- >4 PE likely

[a]Van Belle A, Buller HR, Huisman MV, et al. Effectiveness of managing suspected pulmonary embolism using an algorithm combining clinical probability, D-dimer testing, and computed tomography. JAMA 2006; 295:172.

Symptoms Observed in Patients with PE[a]

	Presentation (%)
Dyspnea	73
Calf or thigh pain	44
Pleuritic pain	44
Calf or thigh swelling	41
Hemoptysis or pleuritic pain	41
Cough	34
Wheezing	21
Chest pain (not pleuritic)	19
Calf and thigh pain	17
Calf and thigh swelling	7

[a]Paul D. Stein (2007) Clinical characteristics of patients with acute pulmonary embolism. Am J Med 120(10): 871–879.

Perfusion defects suspicious for decrease blood flow: Areas of reduce perfusion → cold defects following segmental or subsegmental distribution (Wedge shaped defect) → no perfusion noted distally to the embolus. *Strip sign* is a nonsegmental defect with a layer of perfused lung parenchyma distal to the perfusion defect, likely due to emphysema.

Matched defect (*chronic process*): Ventilation images demonstrate absence of ventilation in the same pattern noted on perfusion images.

Mismatched (*acute process*): Ventilation images demonstrate normal ventilation correspond to poorly perfused segmental defects noted on perfusion images.

Size

1. *Small defect*: less than 25 % of a segment
2. *Moderate defect*: more than 25 % of the segment, and less than 75 % of a segment.
3. *Large defect*: More than 75 % of a segment

Mechanism of Matched and Mismatched Defects

Thrombus within the pulmonary arteries or its brunches → lack of perfusion distal to the embolus (hence segmental/subsegmental/wedge shaped defect is a required criteria) → perfusion dead zone with abnormally increased V/Q ratio (acute mismatched defect) → release of modulators to induce local bronchoconstriction → increase respiratory resistance → regional air flow is reduced (formed ventilation defect) → V/Q ratio is essentially normalized (chronic matched defect). Fast administration of Heparin may dissolve the thrombus and prevent local bronchoconstriction.

False positive results may be noted in patients, which the bronchoconstriction mechanism did not occur. In this case chronic defect may be presented as a stable mismatch defect. Therefore, prior images are needed for the interpretation of VQ scans for patients with known prior PE. Failure of bronchoconstriction may be seen in patients with underlying chronic lung disease or elderly age which bronchial flexibility is altered.

Reading criteria by PIOPAD (prospective), PIOPED II (retrospective), Modified PIOPED II:

Findings	PIOPED	PIOPED II	Modified PIOPED II
No perfusion defects	Normal	Normal	Normal
Non-segmental perfusion defcts (hilum, cardiomegaly, vessels, atelectasis, pacemarekrs, ports, act, etc.) Small pleural effusion Defect smaller than CXR defect 1–3 small defects Strip sign Triple matched defect (in one segment) in upper and middle lobes	Very low probability (<10 % risk for PE)	Low probability (10–19 % risk for PE)	Very low probability (<10 % risk for PE)
1 large or moderate Matched defect* Single moderate size mismatched defect** >3 small defects, normal CXR Moderate size pleural effusion Diffuse heterogeneous perfusion	Low probability (10–19 % risk for PE)		Nondiagnostic
1 large or large equivalent (2 moderate) mismatched defects 1 large or moderate defect in the lower lobes matched by CXR (Triple -Match) Cannot define as high or low probability	Intermediate probability (20–79 % risk for PE)	Intermediate probability (20–79 % risk for PE)	
>2 large (or large equivalents) mismatched defects	High probability (80–100 % risk for PE)	High probability (80–100 % risk for PE)	High probability (80–100 % risk for PE)
≥2 large (or large equivalents)+1 moderate mismatched defects		High probability (100 % risk for PE)	High probability (100 % risk for PE)

*Single moderate size mismatched defect- 36 % cases of PE and **1 Matched defect any size-26 % incident of PE-in POIPED study – hence may be called intermediate probability

Pretest probability and VQ test probability by PIOPED[a]

Scan probability	Clinical probability of emboli			
	High (%)	Moderate (%)	Low (%)	All probabilities (%)
High	96	88	56	87
Intermediate	66	28	16	30
Low	40	16	4	14
Near normal/normal	0	6	2	4
Total	68	30	9	28

[a]PIOPED Investigators (1990) Value of the ventilation/perfusion scan in acute pulmonary embolism. Results of the prospective investigation of pulmonary embolism diagnosis (PIOPED). JAMA 263:2753.

Triple matched [a]

Zone	+PE	−PE	Prevalence of PE (%)
Upper	4	32	11
Middle	6	46	12
Lower	61	126	33
Total	71	204	26

[a]Worsley DF, Kim CK, Alavi A, Palevsky HI (1993) Detailed analysis of patients with matched ventilation/perfusion defects and chest radiographic opacities. J Nucl Med 34:1851–1853

Suggested Reading

- AuntMinnie: Pulmonary Embolism.
- Bronchoconstriction in the Presence of Pulmonary Embolism by V Gurewich (1963) Circulation. XXVII
- Gottschalk A et al (1993) Ventilation-perfusion scintigraphy in the PIOPED study. Part I. Data collection and tabulation. J Nucl Med 34:1109–1118
- Gottschalk A et al (1993) Ventilation-perfusion scintigraphy in the PIOPED study. Part II. Evaluation of the scintigraphic criteria and interpretations. J Nucl Med 34:1119–1126
- Gottschalk A et al (2007) Very low probability interpretation of V/Q lung scans in combination with low probability objective clinical assessment reliability excludes pulmonary embolism. J Nucl Med 48:1411–1415
- Palevsky HI (1991) The problems of the clinical and laboratory diagnosis of pulmonary embolism. Semin Nucl Med 21:276–280
- Stein PD, Gottschalk (1994) Critical review of ventilation/perfusion lung scans in acute pulmonary embolism. Prog Cardiovasc Dis. 37(1):13–24
- Stein PD, Woodard PK, Weg JG et al (2007) Diagnostic pathways in acute pulmonary embolism: recommendations of the PIOPED II Investigators. Radiology 242 (1): 15–21. doi:10.1148/radiol.2421060971
- The PIOPED Investigators (1990) Value of the ventilation/perfusion scan in acute pulmonary embolism. Results of the prospective investigation of pulmonary embolism diagnosis (PIOPED). JAMA 263:2753
- The role of prostaglandins in the bronchoconstriction induced by pulmonary micro-embolism in the guinea-pig (1980). J Physiol 308:427–437
- Worsley DF, Kim CK, Alavi A, Palevsky HI (1993) Detailed analysis of patients with matched ventilation/perfusion defects and chest radiographic opacities. J Nucl Med 34:1851–1853

Distribution and Clearance

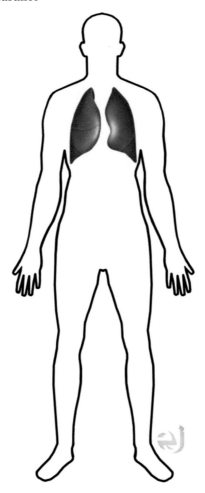

Distribution Pulmonary alveolar capillary bed.
Clearance MAA particles are fragile and will undergo degradation and be phago-cytized in the RES (liver and spleen).

Normal Distribution Patterns

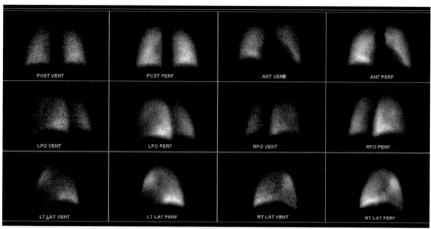

Normal VQ with Tc-99m MAA and Tc-99m DTPA

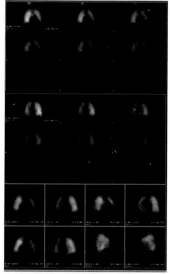

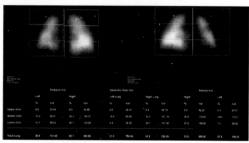

Pre-transplant quantitation evaluation

Normal VQ with Tc-99m MAA (lower
image) and Xe-133 gas (anterior-upper
image, posterior middle image)

Low-Probability VQ Scan

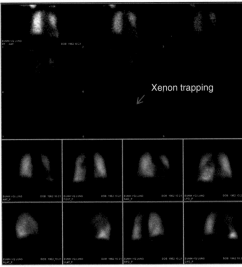

V/Q scan with Xenon: A nonsegmental defect
within the left lung. As well, left upper lobe Xenon
trapping

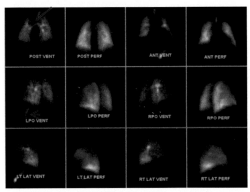

VQ With Tc-99m DTPA. Main bronchial
trapping of Tc-99m DTPA due to COPD (*large
arrow*) and tracer oral ingestion (*small
arrow*)

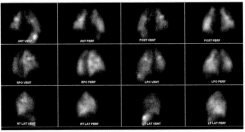

VQ With Tc-99m DTPA. Chronic pulmonary
embolism (multiple bilateral matched defects)

High-Probability VQ Scan

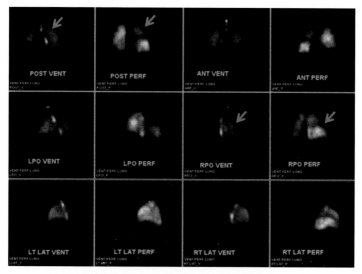

Tc-99m DTPA /Tc-99m MAA VQ scan demonstrates at
least two large mismatched segmental perfusion
defects (absence of perfusion and presence of ventilation)

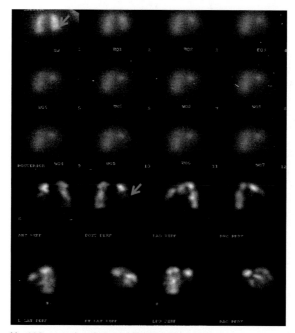

Xe-133 posterior view and Tc-99m MAA VQ
scan demonstrate at least two large
mismatched segmental perfusion defects
within the right inferior lobe

Miscellaneous

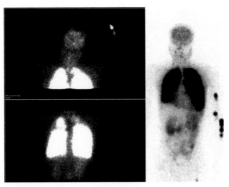

Systemic right-to-left shunt

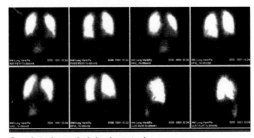

Caudate hepatic lobe is noted
secondary to IVC obstruction

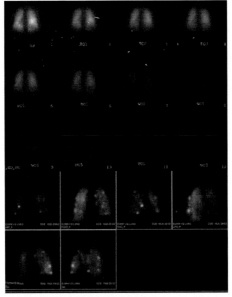

Blood clot formation secondary to
withdrawal of blood into the Tc-99m
MAA syringe with delayed injection

5   Breast

5.1   Tc-99m Sestamibi (MIBI): Molecular Breast Imaging (MBI)

Indication Breast cancer.

Other Uses Cardiac stress scans, parathyroid adenoma.

Tc-99m Generator produced in the form of Tc 99m pertechnetate (TcO_4^{1-}) (+7 valence) from Mo-99. t_{phys} 6 h. *Emits* gamma 140 keV (89 %).

Mechanism *Lipophilic structure:* Passive diffusion to the cell → uptake by mitochondria due to membrane electric potential → retention due to electrostatic interactions → trapped within the mitochondria.

Oxyphil cells: Secreting cell → higher mitochondria concentration → higher tracer retention.

Washout: by Pgp (P glycoprotein). Tumor cell [Pgp] expression is related to tumor multidrug resistance. Can potentially predict chemotherapy tumor resistance (not in use today).

Camera Dedicated breast gamma imaging modalities.

Breast specific gamma camera (BSGI): Single head NaI(Tl) scintillation detector camera for breast-specific gamma imaging.
Molecular breast imaging (MBI): Dual head semisolid-state (CZT) detector camera for molecular breast imaging.

Protocol IV injection of Tc-99m sestamibi. Breast positioning on the camera: similar to mammogram. Bilateral CC, MLO static images for 10 min per position. 10 min × 4 positions = 40 min scan.

Dose 8 mCi.

Image Interpretation According to tailored BI-RAD criteria.

Distribution *Early 30 min:* Thyroid salivary gland, heart >>> liver, kidney.
Late >60 min: Biliary tract, GI, kidney, bladder > liver, heart >> thyroid, salivary gland.

Clearance Bile to GI and kidney.

Recommended Reading
• Michael O'Connor, Deborah Rhodes, Carrie Hruska (2009) Molecular breast imaging. Expert Rev Anticancer Ther 9(8):1073–1080. doi: 10.1586/era.09.75. PMCID: PMC2748346

Distribution and Clearance

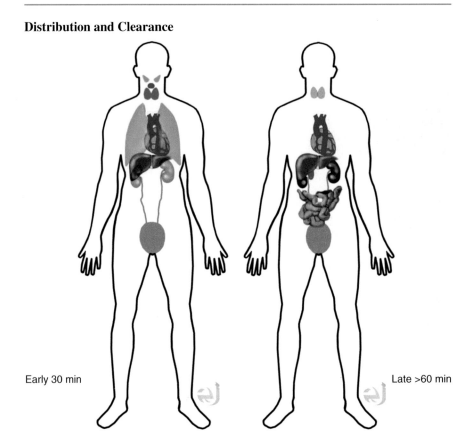

Early 30 min   Late >60 min

Distribution *Early 30 min* Thyroid salivary gland, heart >>> liver, kidney.
   Late >60 min: Biliary tract, GI, kidney, bladder > liver, heart >> thyroid, salivary gland.
Clearance Bile to GI and kidney.

Normal Distribution: Breast

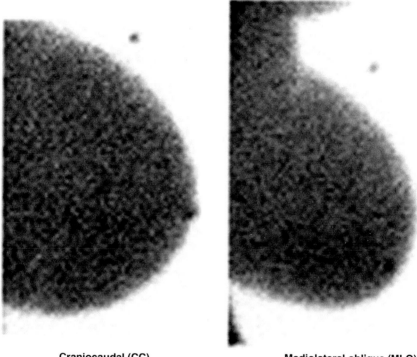

Craniocaudal (CC)   Mediolateral oblique (MLO)

Abnormal Distribution: Breast

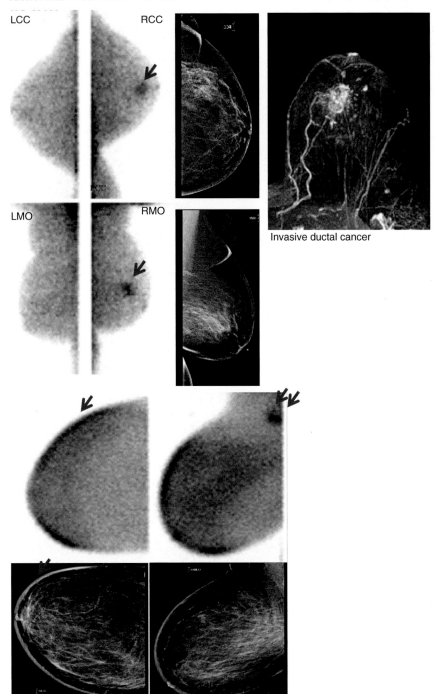

Invasive ductal cancer

Inflammation of the breast–status post trauma (single
arrow). Inflammatory axillary LN (double arrow)

5.2   Ultrafiltered Tc-99m Sulfur Colloid: Lymphoscintigraphy

Indications (1) Oncology – localization of sentinel lymph node (LN) for breast cancer and melanoma. Sentinel lymph node: First LN/LNs group to drain a cancer. (2) Evaluation of lymphedema.

Tc-99m Generator produced in the form of Tc 99m pertechnetate (TcO_4^{1-}) (+7 valence) from Mo-99. t_{phys} 6 h. *Emits* gamma 140 keV (89 %).

Sulfur Colloid Particle size of 0.1–2.0 μm prior to filtration; 0.1–0.2 μm after filtration.

Tc-99m SC Preparation kit *does not include stannous ion* to bind TcO_4^{1-} to SC. The *only* tracer that does not require stannous ion.

Mechanism of Action Subcutaneous/intradermal admin: Tc-99m SC particles will be extracted by subcutaneous lymphatic system (phagocytosis) to regional LNs.

Protocol Tc-99m sulfur colloid boiled for 5 min, cooled for 2 min, and filtered to 0.2 μm. Typical dose: 0.5 mCi.
   melanoma. Intradermal injection into four areas around the lesion.
   Breast CA 4 intradermal/subcutaneous injections: Periareolar, lateral to a surgical scar, palpable mass or in the quadrant where the mass is located.
   Lymphedema: Intradermal or subcutaneous injections within the interphalangeal webs.
   Imaging protocol: Immediate static, 15 min and 30 min postinjection as needed. SPECT/CT may be added for better localization (recommended for head and neck melanoma). For lymphedema image the lower extremities, dynamic or static. Whole body images may be used to investigate the patten of tracer distribution.
   Transmission images: place a large flat source of Co-57 to define the body contours.

Dose Tc-99m sulfur colloid 0.1–1 mCi.

Target Organ Injection site.

Distribution Subcutaneous and lymphedema: SC particles will be extracted by the lymphatic system to regional LNs and continue toward the thoracic duct and the left subclavian vein.

Clearance Via phagocytosis: Tc-99m sulfur colloid particles will be fixed intracellularly.

Distribution Patterns

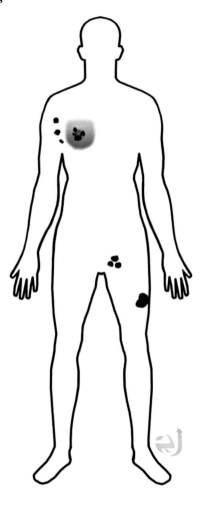

Distribution Subcutaneous: SC particles will be extracted by the lymphatic system to regional LNs.
Clearance Via phagocytosis – Tc-99m sulfur colloid particles will be fixed intracellularly.

5.3   Tc-99m Tilmanocept (Lymphoseek): Lymphoscintigraphy

Indications (1) Oncology- Localization of sentinel lymph node (breast cancer, melanoma). (2) Evaluation of lymphedema.
Sentinel lymph node: First LN/LNs group to drain a cancer.

Tc-99m Generator produced in the form of Tc-99m pertechnetate (TcO_4^{1-}) (+7 valence) from Mo-99. t_{phys} 6 h. *Emits* Gamma 140 KeV (89 %)

Tilmanocept   particle size of 7 nm

Tc-99m Tilmanocept   receptor based tracer targeted CD 206 receptor.

Mechanism of Action   particles will be extracted by intradermal lymphatic system and will be drained to regional LNs → bind to LN phagocytes receptors CD206 for 30 h.

Protocol

Melanoma Intradermal injection into four areas around the lesion.
Breast CA 4 Intradermal injections: periareolar, lateral to a surgical scar, palpable mass or in the quadrant where the mass is located.
Lymphedema: Intradermal injection within the interphalangeal webs.
Image protocol: Immediate, 15 min and 30 min as needed. SPECT/CT may be added for better localization (recommended for head and neck melanoma).
Transmission images: place a large flat source of Cobalt-57 to define the body contours.
Pitfall: Injections should be superficial (intradermal); otherwise failure rate will increase.

Dose   0.5 mCi.

Target Organ   Injection sites.

Distribution   Intradermal: 2–3 min extraction by the subcutaneous lymphatic system to regional LNs.

Clearance   Particles will be fixed within phagocyte receptors CD206.

Distribution Patterns

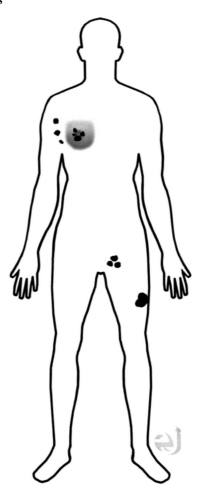

Distribution Tilmanocept Intradermal: 2–3 min extracted by the lymphatic system to regional LNs
Clearance Via phagocytosis – particles will be fixed within phagocyte receptors CD206

Distribution Patterns

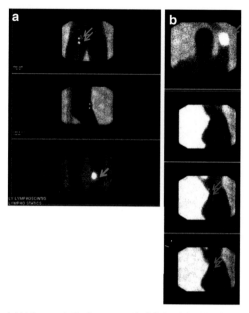

(a) Melanoma in the inner posterior inferior right thigh (arrow) with right inguinal 2 sentinel lymph nodes (double arrow). (b) Melanoma of the left upper extremity with (arrow) 2 sentinel lymph nodes in the axilla

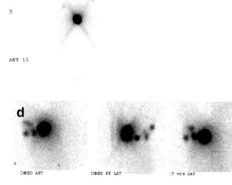

(c) Vulvar Melanoma with bilateral sentinel inguinal lymph nodes (bilateral vulvar injections). (d) Right breast cancer (injection site) with 3 axillary sentinel lymph nodes

6 Heart

6.1 Myocardial Perfusion Scan: MPI

Tracers Rb-82 chloride, TI-201 chloride. Tc-99m tetrofosmin, Tc-99m Sestamibi

Tc-99m Generator produced in the form of Tc-99m pertechnetate (TcO_4^{1-}) from Mo-99. t_{phys} 6 h. *Emits* gamma 140 keV. Image: 20 % window 140 keV peak.

TI-201 Cyclotron produced t_{phys} 73.1 h. *Decays* by electron capture to mercury Hg-201. *Emits* mercury X-ray 69–80 keV (94 %), gamma 135 keV (2.0 %), 167 keV (10 %) *Image:* 20 % window 80 keV peak.

Rb-82 Generator produced from Sr-82/Rb-82 generator system. t_{phys} 76 s *decays* 95 % by positron emission and 5 % by electron capture. *Emits* annihilation photons; gamma ray energy=511 keV, prompt gamma (776 keV, 15 % abundance and 1395 keV 0.5 % abundance). *Image* PET scanner.

First-Pass Extraction

TI-201 (85 %–91 %), Rb-82 (61 %).
Sestamibi (60 %).
Tetrofosmin (50 %).

Total myocardial uptake is up to 2 % of the injected dose for Tc-99m tracers and 5–8 % for Tl-201 and Rb-82.

Mechanism *Tetrofosmin/Sestamibi:* Lipophilic structure. Passive diffusion into the cell → uptake by mitochondria due to membrane electric potential → retention due to electrostatic interactions → trapped within the mitochondria.

Rb-82 Chloride and Tl-201 Chloride Potassium analogs; transport across the myocardial membrane via NA^+-K^+ ATPase.

Viability Scans *Tl-201 – Redistribution:* Dynamic exchange of Tl-201 between circulations to intracellular. Tracer redistribution in a fixed defect → presence of hibernating myocardial tissue → patient will benefit from revascularization.

F-18 FDG viability test (1) Rb-82 rest perfusion protocol (can be done with SPECT tracers also); (2) glucose/insulin load (optional) followed by 10 mCi F-18 FDG; (3) 30 min post-FDG injection, CT, and PET (wait for 60 min for diabetic patients).

Distribution *Tc-99m tetrofosmin*, *Tc-99m sestamibi*: Early (30 min) thyroid salivary gland, heart > heart >>> liver, kidney. Late (60 min) biliary tract, GI, kidney, bladder > liver, heart >> thyroid, salivary gland.

Rb-82 chloride and *Tl-201 chloride*: Proportional to the cardiac output. Five percent coronary arteries, 20 % kidneys. Not crossing BBB.

Clearance *Tc-99m tetrofosmin* and *Tc-99m sestamibi*: Bile to GI and kidney, allows early lung to heart or delayed heart to liver imaging.

Rb-82 chloride and *Tl-201 chloride*: Myocardium, kidneys, thyroid, liver, and stomach.

Distribution and Clearance

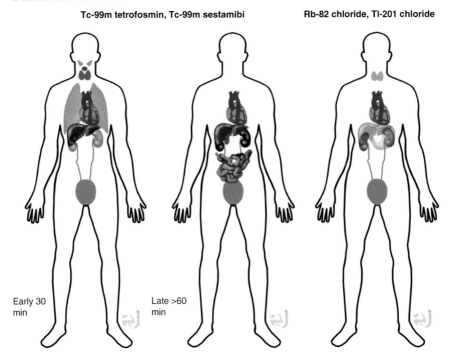

Tc-99m tetrofosmin, Tc-99m sestamibi   **Rb-82 chloride, TI-201 chloride**

Early 30 min   Late >60 min

Distribution

Tc-99m tetrofosmin, Tc-99m sestamibi: Early (30 min) – thyroid salivary gland, heart >>> liver, kidney. Late (>60 min) – biliary tract, GI, kidney, bladder > liver, heart >>>>> thyroid, salivary gland.

TI-201 and *Rb-82*: Proportional to the cardiac output. Five percent coronary arteries, 20 % kidneys. Not crossing BBB.

Clearance

Tc-99m tetrofosmin and *Tc-99m sestamibi*: Bile to GI and kidney, allows early lung to heart or delay heart to liver imaging.

Rb-82 chloride and *Tl-201 chloride*: Myocardium, kidneys, thyroid, liver, and stomach.

6.2 Myocardial Perfusion Scan: MPI Protocols

Preparation Nothing per os (NPO) 2 h. before test, IV line of 18–20 gauge, ECG monitoring into recovery until HR is < 100 bpm. At least 3 min on recovery and all ECG changes have resolved.

Exercise Stress Test *Absolute contraindications:* Unstable angina, decompensated heart failure, BP > 200/110 mmHg, uncontrolled arrhythmias, symptomatic aortic stenosis/dissection, acute PE, acute myocarditis/pericarditis, MI < 4 days, severe pulmonary hypertension.

Relative contraindications: HTOCM (hypertrophic obstructive cardiomyopathy), LBBB (Left bundle branch block), WPW (wolff-parkinson-white) → convert to vasodilators pharmaceuticals.

Protocol: Patients shouldn't take beta-blockers on the morning of the exam. Bruce protocol: 7 stages. Starts at 1.7mph and 10 % grade. Every 3 min treadmill increases incline by 2 % in grade and speed: 1.7, 2.5, 3.4, 4.2, 5.0, 5.5, 6.0 mph. Target HR is 85 % of maximal capacity [(220-age) × (0.85)], or double product (max sys BP x max HR > 25,000). Exercise capacity: normal > 8 min, 20–40 % moderately reduced 6–8 min, <40 % significantly reduced <6 min. Inappropriate response: HR >120 bpm in the first 3 min (deconditioned response), Systolic blood pressure > 220 or Diastolic >115 mmHg during exercise.

Pharmaceutical Stress Test

A. *Dobutamine*: Direct β1 and β2 receptor stimulation → increase heart contractility → increase HR → increase coronary blood flow. t_{biol} of 2 min

   Indication: Patients who can't walk and have severe asthma, COPD or seizures.

   Protocol: infusion starting at dose of 10 mcg/kg/min. Every 3 min increase dose in interval of 10mcg until 50 mcg/kg/min or target HR is achieved. Having patient do isometric exercise during infusion may help increase HR. May give atropine (0.25–0.5 mg, up to 1–2 mg) if target HR is not achieved.

   Absolute Contraindications: same as exercise.

   Termination: Stop infusion after Tc-99 injection. If necessary may reverse the effects with beta blockade; example: metoprolol 5 mg IV push.

B. *Vasodilators*: A2a receptor activators → coronary vasodilation (areas of calcification will not be dilated appropriately and resulting in hypoperfused myocardium).

Hemodynamic effect: Increase in HR and decrease in BP.

Common side effects: Chest pain, shortness of breath, Headache (most common), flushing, nausea, dyspnea, dizziness, and hypotension. Side effects may be reversed with aminophylline 50–100 mg IV, may push up to 300 mg for severe side effects.

Indication: Handicap, LBBB, WPW, post-MI 1–4 days.

1. *Adenosine*: Nonselective activation or A2a receptors. Other receptor activation: A2b and A3 (bronchospasm), A1 (AV block), A2b (peripheral vasodilation).

   Protocol: infusion of 140 mg/kg/min for 6 min with IV radiopharmaceutical injection at the 3 min point of the infusion of adenosine prior to termination (gamma/PET agent).

Absolute contraindications: Asthmatic patients with active wheezing, 2nd and 3rd AV block without pacemaker, SBP<90, recent use of dipyridamole/dipyridamole-containing medications, < 24 h use of caffeine or aminophylline, acute MI.

Relative contraindications: HR<40 bpm.

Termination: stop infusion ($t_{1/2}$ <10 s).

2. *Regadenoson*: Selective activation of A2a receptor. Minimal to none A1, A2b, and A3. $t_{1/2}$ 2–4 min.

   Protocol: IV push of 0.4 mg over 10–15 s followed by radiopharmaceutical (gamma/PET agent).

   Absolute contraindications: Asthmatic patients with active wheezing (controversial), 2nd and 3rd AV block without pacemaker, SBP<90, recent use of dipyridamole or dipyridamole-containing medications, caffeine, or aminophylline within 24 h, acute MI, seizure history.

   Relative contraindications: HR<40 bpm.

   Termination: Give aminophylline 100 mg if needed for side effects.

3. *Dipyridamole*: Indirect coronary vasodilator. Plasma protein bound that prevents reuptake and deamination of adenosine.

   Protocol: Infusion of 0.142 mg/kg/min or 0.56 mg/kg for 4 min, wait for 3 min then inject radiopharmaceutical IV.

   Absolute and relative contraindications: Same as adenosine.

   Termination: Stop the infusion and give aminophylline 100 mg if needed for side effects. ($T_{1/2}$ varies for different receptors).

Myocardial Perfusion Protocols

Two day protocol stress/rest

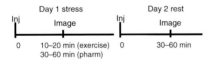

Same day protocol rest/stress with TI 201/Tc-99m

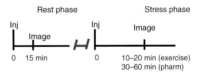

Same day protocol stress/rest Tc-99m/Tc-99m

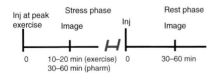

⊢ 3:1 Tc-99m dose ratio: Wait for 2 h.
3.5–4:1 Tc-99m ratio: no waiting time is necessary
Inj: Injection

Same day protocol rest/ stress with Tc-99m/Tc-99m

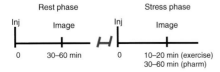

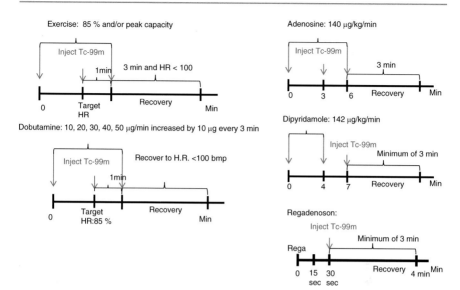

Pitfalls

- Cardiac PET images using Rb-82 are done simultaneously with the pharmaceutical injection due to Rb-82 short Tphys of 75 s.
- Adenosine has shorter t_{biol} than dipyridamole. Patients are more symptomatic (SOB, nausea, and discomfort) when stressed with dipyridamole.
- Aminophylline will reverse the effect of regadenoson and dipyridamole. Cup of coffee will have the same effect.
- Aminophylline and regadenoson may lower seizure threshold in patients with a history of seizures.

Suggested Reading

Henzlova et al. ASNC imaging guidelines for nuclear cardiology procedures. Stress protocols and tracers. J Nucl Cardiol 1071–3581. doi:10.1007/s12350-009-9062-4

6.3   Myocardial Perfusion Scan: Interpretation

Defect Size Small – 10 % of the entire myocardium. Medium – 10–20 %. Large – >20 %.

Location *Basal* (segments 1–6): *1* – anterior, *2* – anteroseptal, *3* – inferoseptal, *4* – inferior, *5* – inferolateral, *6* – anterolateral. *Mid* (segments 7–12): *7* – anterior, *8* – anteroseptal, *9* – inferoseptal, *10* – inferior *11* – inferolateral, *12* – anterolateral. *Apical* (segments 13–17): *13* – anterior, *14* – septal, *15* – inferior, *16* – lateral, *17* – apex.

Coronary Artery *Left anterior descending (LAD)*: Diagonal branches supply the anterior wall and the septal branches supply the septum. *Right coronary artery (RCA)*: Supplies the right ventricle and basal septum. Eighty percent of the RCA gives the posterior descending artery (PDA) branch (right dominant) which supplies the inferior and inferolateral wall. *Left circumflex (LCX)*: Supplies the lateral wall via the obtuse marginal (OM) artery, and in 20 % of population LCX will give branch to PDA and supply inferior wall. Additional variant: 10 % PDA will be codominant.

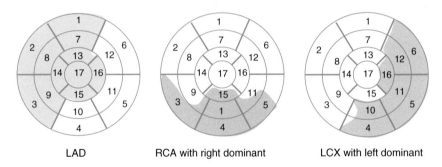

LAD   RCA with right dominant   LCX with left dominant

Severity >3SD (standard deviations) counts below normal population → defect on the polar map.

Summed Stress Score (SSS) Accumulative score for severity for each segment (0–4) 0 – normal, 1 – mild reduction, 2 – moderate reduction, 3 – severe reduction, 4 – absent of counts. The summed rest score (SRS) is similar scoring system for rest images. The summed difference score (SDS) defines level of reversibility of defect between stress and rest = SSS-SRS.

SSS: Normal < 4, moderate = 9–13, severe > 13.

SDS: No ischemia < 2, mild ischemia = 2–4, moderate ischemia = 5–8, severe ischemia > 8.

Suggested Reading
- Hachamovitch R, Berman DS, Shaw LJ et al (1998) Incremental prognostic value of myocardial perfusion single-photon emission computed tomography for the prediction of cardiac death: differential stratification for risk of cardiac death and myocardial infarction. Circulation 97:535–543

MPI

Diaphragmatic attenuation

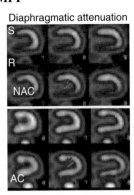

Breast attenuation

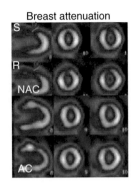

LAD infarct

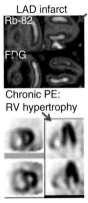

Chronic PE:
RV hypertrophy

Ischemia

LCX   RCA   LAD

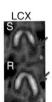   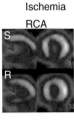   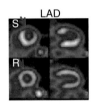

False positive due to LBBB

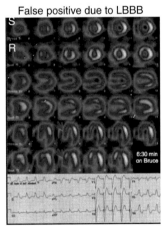

Viability scan-viable myocardium
at the LAD distribution

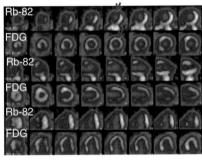

6.4   Multiple-Gated Acquisition (MUGA)

Indications Prechemotherapy evaluation of ejection fraction (EF); evaluation of EF secondary to abnormal cardiac function tests.

Tc-99m Generator produced in the form of Tc 99m pertechnetate (TcO_4^{1-}) (+7 valence) from Mo-99 generator.

Tagging RBC *In vivo* labeling efficiency 75–80 %. *Modified in vivo [in vitro]* labeling efficiency 85–90 %. *In vitro* labeling efficiency >97 %.

Biological Half-Life 24–30 h.

Mechanism

In the blood tube, TcO_4^{1-} reduced intracellularly from +7 to +4 (by stannous) → bind intracellular protein (Hgb ß-globin chain) in the red blood cell.

Dose *Adults:* 15–30 mCi. *Pediatrics:* 0.2–0.4 mCi/kg with a minimum dose of 2–4 mCi.

Protocol *Imaging* EKG strip to evaluate sinus rhythm. Position the detector in the LAO projection → acquire R-R interval gated images for at least 16 frames/cycle. For better performance and accuracy, increase to 32–64 frames/cycle (other frame # are being used as well).

Image processing: Region of interest (ROI) around the left ventricle. As well as background (BKG) crescent shape ROI at 4–5 o'clock at the space between the spleen and the left ventricle. Software calculates the sum counts of each frame → *end-diastolic volume* (*EDV*): Frame with the highest counts. *End-systolic volume* (*ESV*): Frame with the lowest counts.

$$EF = \frac{\left(\text{End-diastolic counts-BKG counts}\right) - \left(\text{End-systolic counts-BKG counts}\right)}{\left(\text{End-diastolic counts-BKG counts}\right)}$$

Fourier Phase Analysis Demonstrates inphase and out of phase of the R-R cycle within the ventricle. Normally, both ventricles are out of phase to the atria.

Phase Histogram Will demonstrate beat-to-beat contractility. Normally should be high and narrow. If low peak → contractility is decreased. If wide → intra- and interventricular dyssynchrony (e.g., aneurysm, LBBB).

Interpretation Normal EF 50–75 %.

Critical Organ Heart.

Pitfall EF will increase if BKG placed on high count regions – such as the spleen or the aorta.

Distribution Aorta and its branches, liver, and heart.

Abnormal Distribution Free Tc will be taken up by the thyroid, salivary glands, gastric mucosa, and bowel.

Clearance Decay and renal.

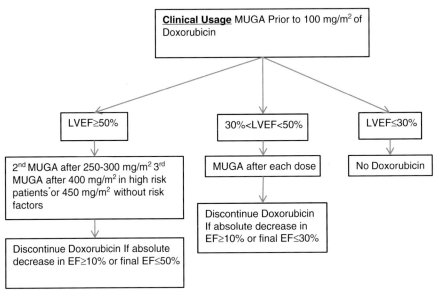

*High risk: abnormal ECG, heart disease, prior radiation exposure, cyclophosphamide therapy, or cumulative dose already >450 mg/m^2.

Suggested Reading
- Schwartz RG et al. (1987) Congestive heart failure and left ventricular dysfunction complicating doxorubicin therapy. Seven-year experience using serial radionuclide angiocardiography. Am J Med. 82(6):1109–1118
- Society of Nuclear Medicine Procedure Guideline for Gated Equilibrium Radionuclide Ventriculography version 3.0, approved June 15, 2002

Distribution and Clearance

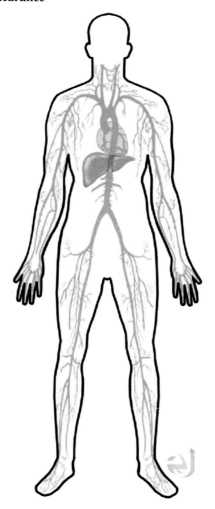

Distribution Aorta and its branches, liver, and heart.
Clearance Decay and elimination via kidneys.

MUGA: Normal

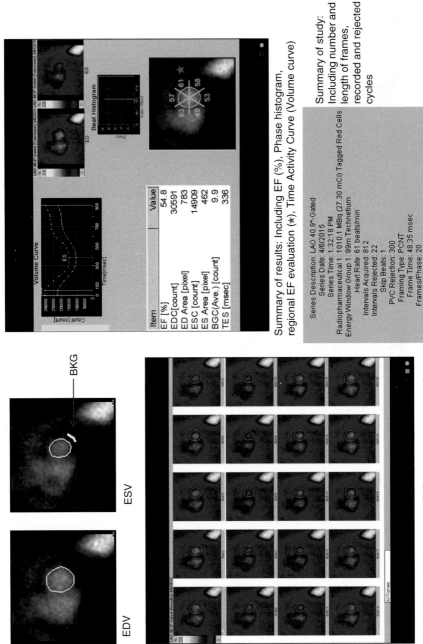

Summary of results: Including EF (%), Phase histogram, regional EF evaluation (★), Time Activity Curve (Volume curve)

Summary of study: Including number and length of frames, recorded and rejected cycles

Series Description: LAO 40.9°-Gated
Series Date: 4/6/2015
Series Time: 1:32:18 PM
Radiopharmaceutical 1: 1010.1 MBq (27.30 mCi) Tagged Red Cells
Energy Window Group 1: 99m Technetium
Heart Rate: 61 beats/min
Intervals Acquired: 812
Intervals Rejected: 22
Skip Beats: 1
PVC Rejection: 300
Framing Type: PCNT
Frame Time: 48.35 msec
Frames/Phase: 20

Item	Value
EF [%]	54.8
EDC[count]	30591
ED Area [pixel]	783
ESC [count]	14909
ES Area [pixel]	462
BGC(Ave.) [count]	9.9
TES [msec]	336

BKG

EDV

ESV

Sum images of 20 frames per R-R interval cycle protocol

MUGA: Abnormal

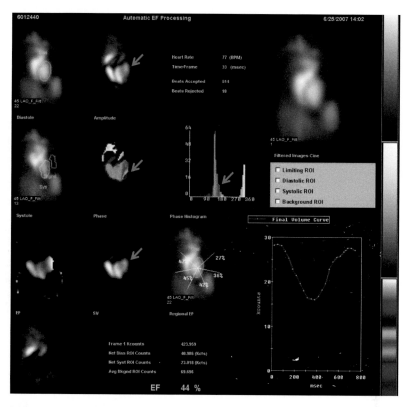

Left ventricular aneurysm: Beat Phase image and histogram demonstrate in-phase and out-of phase colors within the ventricle, characteristic of paradoxical motion secondary to aneurysm.

7   Liver and Spleen

7.1 Tc-99m Mebrofenin (Choletec) or Tc99m Disofenin (Hepatolite): "HIDA Study"

Indications Acute cholecystitis, biliary leak, biliary atresia (neonatal).

Tc-99m Generator produced in the form of Tc-99m pertechnetate (TcO_4^1) from Mo-99. t_{phys} 6 h. *Emits* gamma 140 keV (89 %).

HIDA Hepatobiliary iminodiacetic acid.

Mebrofenin (BrIDA, Choletec) or Disofenin (IDA, iminodiacetic acid) Radiopharmaceutical. Dimer complex. IDA structure is similar to lidocaine (developed as heart-imaging agent).

Mechanism Same pathway as bilirubin: IV injection → bound to plasma protein (mainly albumin) → liver (space of Disse) dissociates from the proteins → hepatocytes (same as the enterohepatic circulation) → transported into bile canaliculi (active transport) unmetabolized.

Protocol *Preparation*: Obtain last meal time (inpatient: clear diet is not a fat-containing meal). NPO 3–4 h prior to scan (ensure gallbladder is not contracted). If NPO more than 24 h, likely gallbladder (GB) is full (sludge), give cholecystokinin (CCK) to empty GB. Wait 30 min after injection. Hold narcotics for at least 6 h prior to scan.

Imaging Upper abdomen, flow 1 s × 60 s → dynamic 1 min × 60 min.

Critical Organ Bowel.
   Acute cholecystitis: Schema A.
   Bile leak: Suspicious extravasation → obtained delayed images including pelvis and surgical drain bag (as needed) up to 24 (may add SPECT/CT for localization).
   Biliary atresia: IV phenobarbital (5mg/kg/day for 5 days) → abdominal images → if no bowel → 24 h delay images.

Dose *Adults:* kit IV injection 5–10 mCi.

Dose Adjustment
Bilirubin <2 mg/dl: 5 mCi.
Bilirubin 2–10 mg/dl: 7.5 mCi.
Bilirubin >10 mg/dl-10 mCi.

   Children: 0.2 mCi/kg (min of 1 mCi).

EF Protocol

1. *Oral fat-containing meal* (i.e., Ensure).
2. *IV infusion of CCK* 0.02 μg/kg for 30 min or 0.01 μg/kg for 60 min.

Imaging for 60 min (dynamic) – calculate EF (N > ~34–38 %).

Distribution Hepatic uptake 98 % (11 min postinjection). GB (10–15 min postinjection).

Clearance Bowel (30–60 min postinjection); renal excretion: 1 % (first 3 h).

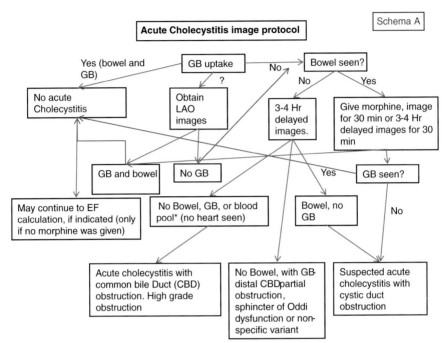

*If Blood pool is seen with no GB or Bowel at 24 h – suspect liver dysfunction

Distribution and Clearance

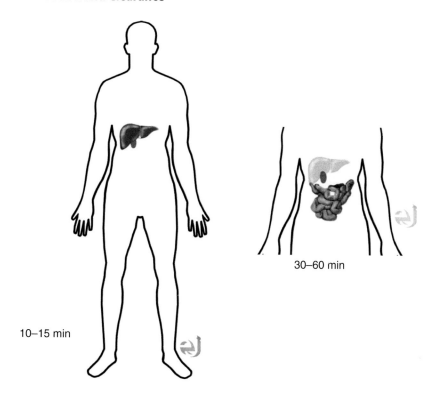

10–15 min

30–60 min

Distribution Hepatic uptake 98 % (11 min postinjection). GB (10–15 min postinjection).

Clearance Bowel (30–60 min postinjection), renal excretion: 1 % (first 3 h).

Normal Distribution

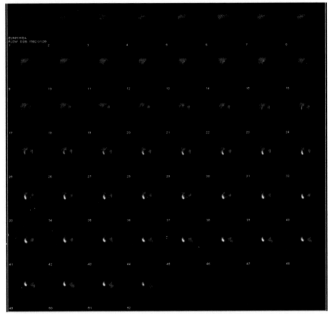

Normal distribution: Immediate hepatic uptake. Gallbladder
and bowel loops are visualized at 10 –15 min post injection.

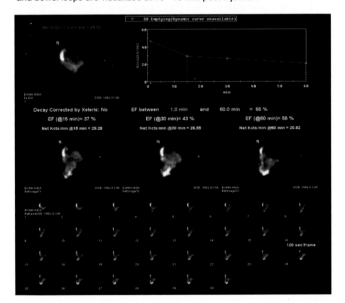

EF calculation after fatty meal or CCK: Rapid contraction of GB
with EF> 34 %–38 %.

Abnormal Distribution

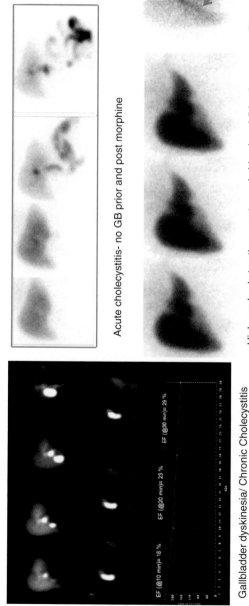

Acute cholecystitis- no GB prior and post morphine

Gallbladder dyskinesia/ Chronic Cholecystitis –low EF (< 34 %)

EF (@10 min)= 16 %

EF (@20 min)= 23 %

EF (@30 min)= 29 %

High-grade obstruction – no tracer in blood pool (blood pool residual is typical for liver dysfunction), and no liver to bowel transition.

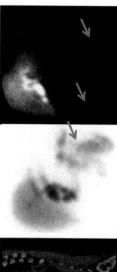

Rim sign- may suggest gangrenous cholecystitis

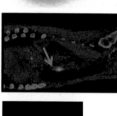

Biliary leak

Fulminant liver- Budd-Chiari syndrome – High blood tracer residual with time

7.2   Liver-Spleen: Tc-99m Sulfur Colloid (SC): IV Injection

Indication Evaluation of liver function. Diagnosis of focal nodular hyperplasia. Evaluation for splenosis. Bone marrow (BM) imaging – evaluation of BM reticuloendothelial system (RES) to diagnose osteomyelitis and avascular necrosis.

Tc-99m Generator produced in the form of Tc 99m pertechnetate (TcO_4^{1-}) (+7 valence) from Mo-99. t_{phys} 6 h. *Emits* gamma 140 keV (89 %).

Sulfur Colloid Particle size of 0.1–2.0 µm (not filtered).

Tc-99m SC Preparation kit *does not include stannous ion* to bind TcO_4^{1-} with SC – the *only* Tc-99m tracer that does not require stannous ion.

Mechanism of Action SC particles will be taken up via phagocytosis to the RES (liver Kupfer cells, macrophages in lymph nodes, BM, and spleen) and will be trapped. Alteration in normal macrophage distribution will result in abnormal scan.

Protocol Inject Tc-99m sulfur colloid intravenously. Twenty minutes after injection, planar images of the abdomen in multiple projections. SPECT images can be added as needed. Bone marrow images – perform in conjunction with WBC scan. Perform planar images.

Dose 1–8 mCi (typical dose: 5 mCi).

Target Organ Liver.

Interpretation *Normal scan*: <u>Liver spleen:</u> Liver uptake > spleen >> homogenous uptake within the red BM (age based). *Abnormal scan* : <u>Liver spleen:</u> Colloid shift – spleen uptake > liver. <u>Bone marrow scan:</u> Mismatch with WBC scans – Tc-99m WBCs demonstrate increase uptake, while Tc-99m SC demonstrates no uptake within the bone marrow due to marrow infiltration with inflammatory cells and edema → obstructs blood flow to BM small arterioles. <u>FNH:</u> hyperplasia of hepatocytes → increase Kupfer cells → increased uptake compared with background.

Distribution 85 % liver Kupfer cells (phagocytes), spleen macrophages (10 %), and bone marrow (5 %).

Clearance IV via phagocytosis – Tc-99m sulfur colloid particles will be fixed intracellularly.

Distribution Patterns

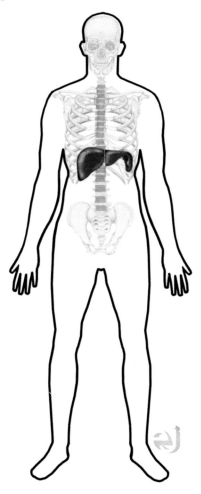

Distribution 85 % liver Kupfer cells (phagocytes), spleen macrophages (10 %), and bone marrow (5 %).
Clearance Via phagocytosis – Tc-99m sulfur colloid particles will be fixed intracellularly.

Normal Distribution Patterns

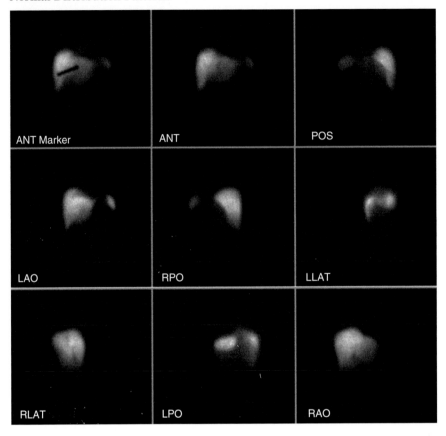

Patient with chronic anemia. Increased uptake by the bone marrow

Abnormal Distribution Patterns

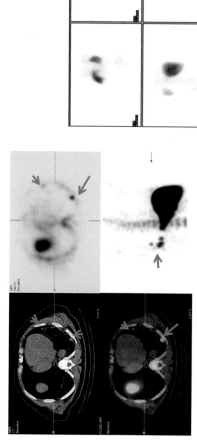

Lung splenosis. Patient underwent spleen resection and diaphragmatic repair

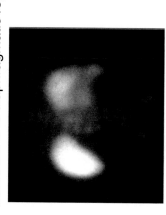

Colloid shift: spleen uptake>>>liver with significant bone marrow uptake

8   Gastrointestinal

8.1   Tc-99m Sulfur Colloid: Oral Gastric Emptying

Indications Gastroparesis.

Tc-99m Generator produced in the form of Tc-99m pertechnetate (TcO_4^{1-}) (+7 valence) from Mo-99. t_{phys} 6 h. *Emits* gamma 140 keV (89 %).

Sulfur Colloid Particle size of 0.1–2.0 μm.

Tc-99m SC Preparation kit *does not include stannous ion* to bind TcO_4^{1-} with SC – the *only* Tc-99m tracer that does not require stannous ion.

Protocol

Solid meal: Tc-99m SC added to 4 oz egg white cooked into scrambled egg (dedicated microwave can be used). Add two slices of toasted white bread, 30 g strawberry jam, and 120 mL water. Should be ingested within 10–15 min.
Semisolid: Oatmeal mixed with hot water and Tc-99m SC.

Imaging

Solid meal: Spot images at 0, 60, 120, 180, 240 min; residual food will be calculated using geometric mean.
Semisolids: Dynamic images for 90 min. $t_{1/2}$ of emptying will be calculated using geometric mean (correct attenuation error).

$$\text{Geometric Mean} = \sqrt{\text{Anterior cts} \times \text{Posterior cts}}$$

Mechanism of Action SC particles will strongly bind to the exposed albumin in egg white.

Dose 0.5–1.0 mCi.

Target Organ Large intestine.

Normal Scan *Solid*: Residual < 10 % at any time point. *Semisolid*: $t_{1/2}$ of emptying should be < 75 min (no consensus).

Distribution GI tract.

Clearance Fecal excretion.

Distribution Patterns

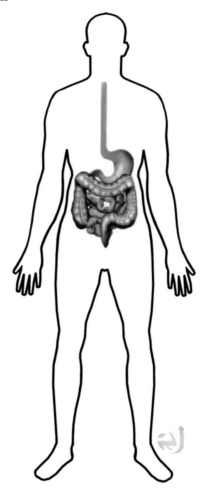

Distribution GI tract.
Clearance Fecal excretion.

Normal vs. Abnormal Distribution Pattern

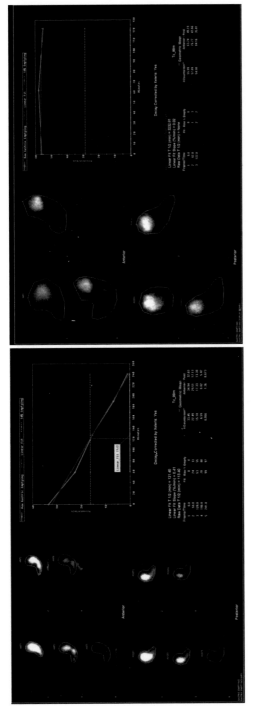

Normal gastric emptying

Abnormal gastric emptying

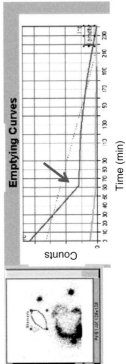

Rapid gastric emptying – may suggest dumping syndrome

8.2 Tagged RBC, GI Bleed Scan

Indications GI bleeds, other bleeding sites.

Other Indications Liver hemangiomas and MUGA.

Tc-99m Generator produced in the form of Tc-99m pertechnetate (TcO_4^{1-}) (+7 valence) from Mo-99. t_{phys} 6 h. *Emits* gamma 140 keV (89 %).

Tagging *In vivo* labeling efficiency 75–80 %. *Modified in vivo* [*in vitro*] labeling efficiency 85–90 %. *In vitro* with Ultratag kit: labeling efficiency >97 %.

Mechanism In the red blood cell, TcO_4^{1-} reduced intracellularly from +7 to +4 (by stannous) → bind intracellular protein (Hgb, beta chain). *Detection* 2–3 cc of blood, rates as low as 0.05–0.1 ml/min.

Imaging *Flow* 1 s × 60 s → *dynamic* 1 min × 60 min → continue to 90 min if negative or inconclusive → may scan for additional 30 min, if still inconclusive → *static* obtain laterals (bladder vs. rectal bleeding) → *delayed static or dynamic* can be done at 2–4 h.

Positive Criteria (1) Appearance of new activity. (2) Increase in intensity over time (3) Antegrade and/or retrograde motion (intraluminal).

Delay Images Confirm GI bleeding if positive, will not localize origin of bleeding due to interval gravity, unless follow positive criteria under dynamic images.

Critical Organ Heart.

Distribution Aorta and its branches, liver, and heart.
Abnormal distribution: Free pertechnetate will be taken up by thyroid, salivary glands, gastric mucosa, and bowel.

Clearance Decay and renal.

Pitfalls

False-positive uptake: Ileal conduit urine uptake, penile "blush" (men with nocturnal erection), Foley catheter urine secretion.
Heparinized patients, patients undergoing blood transfusion, and patients on chemotherapy within last 7–10 days: Expect interference with labeling efficiency.

Distribution and Clearance

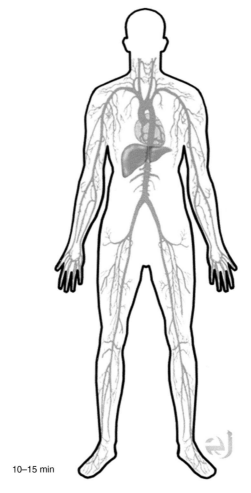

10–15 min

Distribution Aorta and its branches, liver, and heart.
Clearance Decay and renal.

Normal Distribution

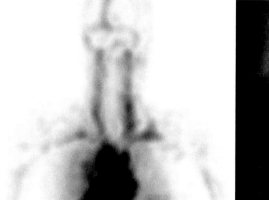 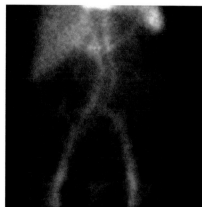

Distribution Aorta and its branches, liver, and heart.
Clearance Blood pool decay and renal.

Abnormal Distribution

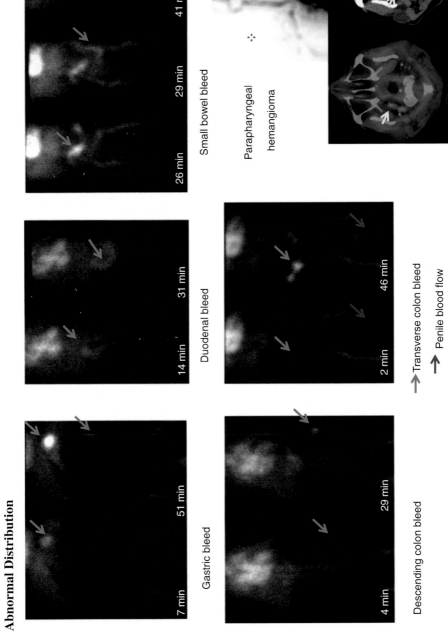

Small bowel bleed

Parapharyngeal hemangioma

Duodenal bleed

Gastric bleed

Transverse colon bleed
Penile blood flow

Descending colon bleed

8.3   Meckel's Diverticulum Scan

Tc-99m Perchnetate: Generator produced. Molybdenum-99 (Mo-99). *Generator* (half-life of 66 h) elutes Tc-99m pertechnetate daughter (TcO_4^{1-}). t_{phys} 6 h. *Emits* gamma 140 keV (89 %).

Meckel's Diverticulum Ectopic gastric mucosa that might bleed.

Mechanism Tc-99m pertechnetate will be rapidly absorbed and secreted by mucus cells of the gastric mucosa. Rapid gastric uptake will be noted. In the presence of gastric mucosa within a Meckel's diverticulum, an area of Tc-99m (TcO_4^{1-}) uptake will be seen. H2 blocker prior to the exam → minimized abnormal secretion of tracer by the gastric mucosa → decreased accumulation of tracer in gastric mucosa → decrease false positive.

Protocol <u>Patient preparation:</u> Fasting 4 h prior. Crushed cimetidine 30 min prior to the exam.

5–10 mg/kg/day or 1.2–2.5 mg/kg orally for children
300 mg for adults.

Dose Children – 30–100 µCi/kg (minimum of 200 µCi). Adults – 10 mCi.

Imaging 1 min flow (60, 1 s/frame). Static images every 5–10 min for 1 h or dynamic images with image every 60 s × 60 min.

Interpretation Positive study will demonstrate an ectopic focus of increased uptake in the abdomen. *False positive* Kidneys, collecting system, and washed stomach mucosal uptake.

Distribution and Clearance

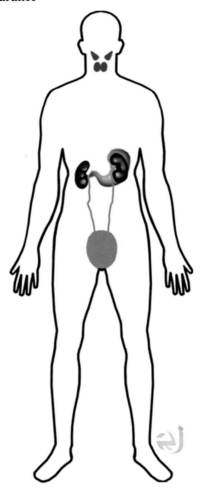

Distribution Thyroid, salivary gland, stomach, and kidney.
Clearance Kidneys → bladder.

Normal Distribution

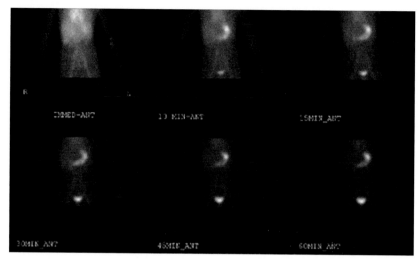

Normal distribution of Tc-99m (TcO_4^{1-}).

Abnormal Distribution

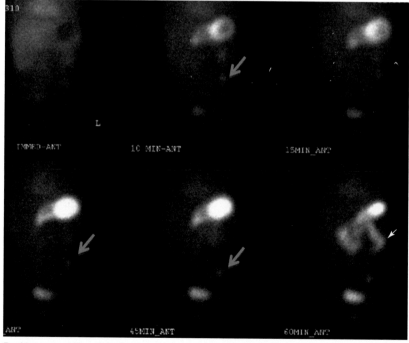

Positive scan with uptake in an ectopic gastric mucosa within the left lower abdomen in a young child (blue arrows), stable in location throughout the study. If motion is noted –will support GI contamination from gastric tracer secretion or active GI bleeding (white arrow).

9   Neuroendocrine

9.1   Indium-111 OctreoScan (In-111 Pentetreotide)

Indications Neuroendocrine tumor localization: SSTR 2 and 5 density based carcinoid tumors, gastrinoma, paraganglioma > pheochromocytoma and neuroblastoma > insulinoma >> medullary thyroid carcinoma.

In-111 Cyclotron produced t_{phys} 2.83 days (67 h). *Emits* gamma rays: 173 (89 %) and 247 (94 %) keV.

Pentetreotide Octreotide + diethylenetriaminepentaacetic acid (DTPA).

Mechanism Via human somatostatin receptors SSTR1-5, pentetreotide will attach to SSTR2 = SSTR5 >>> SSTR3 not to SSTR1 and SSTR4.

Protocol *Preparation:* Bowel preparation, stop octreotide acetate therapy for 24 h prior for short-acting drugs and 4–6 weeks for long-acting drugs.
Scan at 4 h whole-body planar images + SPECT/CT of region of interest → if scan is negative or inconclusive: continue with whole-body and SPECT/CT (as needed) at 24 h.

Dose *Adults:* 6 mCi, *Pediatrics:* 0.14 mCi/Kg.

Image *Photopeak:* 20 % window around 173 and 247 keV; *Collimator:* Low energy.

Critical Organ Spleen.

Distribution

4 h spleen > kidneys, bladder, liver >>> thyroid gland, gallbladder >>> blood pool (10 %).
24 h target (better target to background ratio) > = spleen, kidney > liver > bowel >>> thyroid gland, gallbladder, bladder.

Clearance Rapidly cleared by the kidneys, 2 % hepatobiliary.

Distribution and Clearance

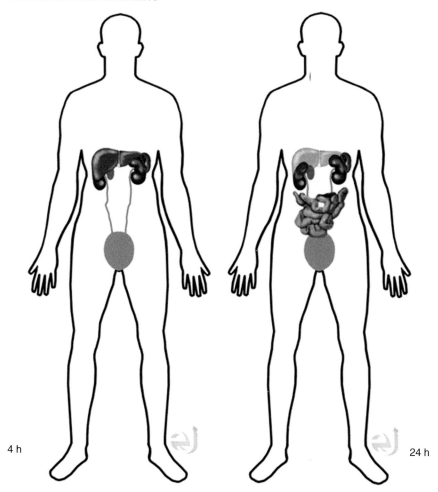

4 h   24 h

Distribution

4 h spleen > kidneys, bladder, liver >>> thyroid gland, gallbladder >>> blood pool (10 %).

24 h target (better target to background ratio) > = spleen, kidney > liver > bowel >>> thyroid gland, gallbladder, bladder.

Clearance Rapidly cleared by the kidneys, 2 % hepatobiliary.

Normal Distribution

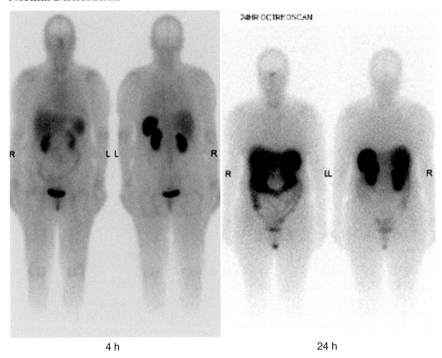

4 h   24 h

Distribution
4 h spleen>kidneys, bladder, liver >>> thyroid gland, gallbladder >>> blood pool
(10 %).

24 h target (better target to background ratio) > = spleen, kidney > liver > bowel
>>> thyroid gland, gallbladder, bladder.

Clearance Rapidly cleared by the kidneys, 2 % hepatobiliary.

Carcinoid Distribution Patterns

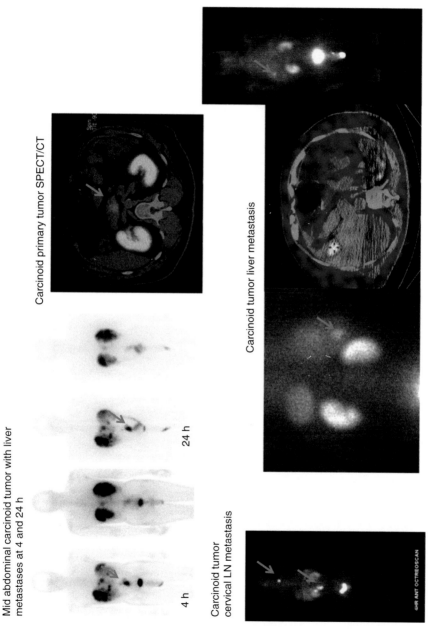

Mid abdominal carcinoid tumor with liver metastases at 4 and 24 h

4 h

24 h

Carcinoid primary tumor SPECT/CT

Carcinoid tumor cervical LN metastasis

Carcinoid tumor liver metastasis

NET: Distribution Patterns

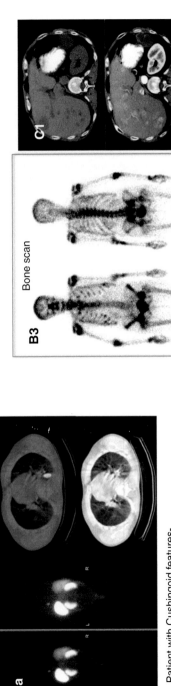

a. Patient with Cushingoid features-
Octreoscan demonstrate ectopic Lung
ACTH producing NET.

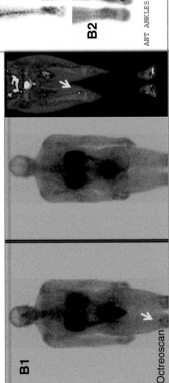

VIPoma: CT (c.1) and
Octreoscn (c.2)

2 cases of Somatostatin receptor avid- Mesenchymal tumor (*yellow arrows*) produce
Phosphotonin seen on Octreoscan (b1and b2.) → phosphorus loss → Osteomalacia seen on
bone scan (b3.).

9.2   Gallium-68 DOTA-Conjugated Peptides

Indications Localization of neuroendocrine tumor (NET), expressing somatostatin receptors (SSTR). *In Europe*: May be used to determine feasibility for Lu-177 or Y-90-DOTA-peptide radionuclide treatment.

Ga-68 *Production*: Ge-68/Ga-68 generator. Ge-68 (Germanium), with half-life of 271 days → Ga-68 (Gallium) with half-life of 68 min. *Decays*: β+(PET tracer).

DOTA Tetraazacyclododecane-tetraacetic acid, the chelator for the peptides TATE, TOC, NOC.

Mechanism *Attached* via human somatostatin receptors SSTR1-5, octreotide (PolyPeptide) will bind to SSTR according to affinity.

Ga-68-DOTA-TATE (FDA orphan drug designation): Ga-68-DOTA0-Tyr(3)-octreotate: predominant affinity only to SSTR2.

Ga-68-DOTA-NOC Ga-68-DOTA0-1-NaI(3)-octreotide: SSRT 2 >>> 3, 5.

Ga-68-DOTA-TOC Ga-68-DOTA0-Tyr(3)-octreotide: SSTR 2 >>> 5.

Protocol
Preparation: Bowel preparation, stop octreotide acetate therapy for 24 h prior for short-acting drugs and 4–6 weeks for long-acting drugs.

Dose 3–8 mCi. Average of 5 mCi.
Scan: At 45 min postinjection for Ga-68-DOTA-TATE or 60–90 min for NOC or TOC.
Dose: 6 mCi.

Critical Organ Spleen.

Distribution *According to the presence of SSTR receptors and affinity*. Spleen> kidneys, pituitary, adrenals >>liver>>> thyroid gland, bladder >>> blood pool.
Pitfall: Pancreatic uncinate process/head has high concentration of SSTR 2. With the high PET resolution normal physiological uptake is commonly seen → may result in a false-positive read.

Clearance Rapidly cleared by the kidneys, 2 % hepatobiliary.

Reference
Virgolini I (2013). Procedure guidelines for PET/CT tumor imaging with Ga-68-DOTA- conjugated peptides: Ga-68-DOTA-TOC, Ga-68-DOTA-NOC, Ga-68-DOTA-TATE. Eur J Nucl Med Mol Imaging 37(10):2004–2010

Distribution and Clearance

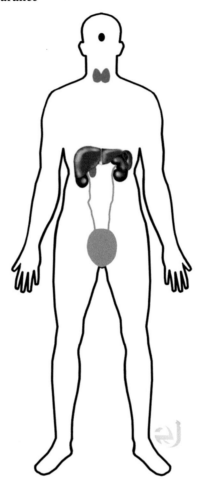

Distribution *According to the presence of SSTR receptors and affinity:* Spleen > kidneys, pituitary, adrenals >> liver >>> thyroid gland, bladder >>> blood pool.
Clearance Rapid renal clearance, 2 % hepatobiliary.

Normal Distribution

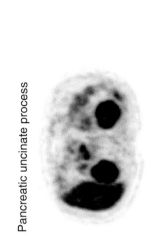

Pancreatic uncinate process

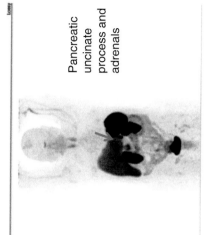

Pancreatic uncinate process and adrenals

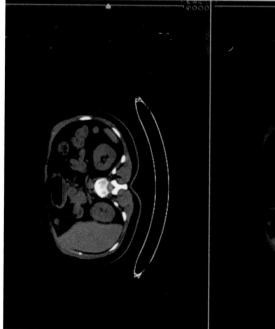

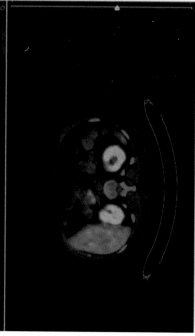

Distribution Patterns: Abnormal

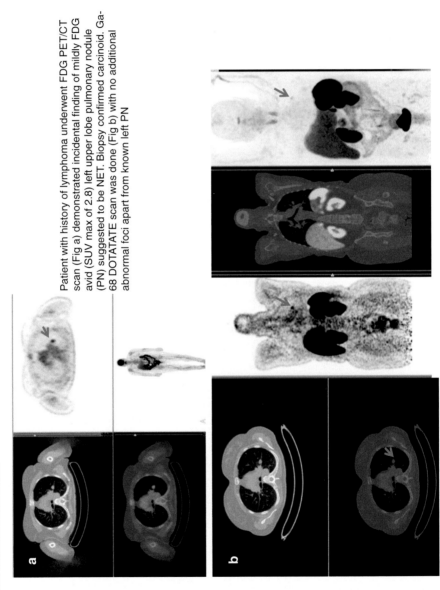

Patient with history of lymphoma underwent FDG PET/CT scan (Fig a) demonstrated incidental finding of mildly FDG avid (SUV max of 2.8) left upper lobe pulmonary nodule (PN) suggested to be NET. Biopsy confirmed carcinoid. Ga-68 DOTATATE scan was done (Fig b) with no additional abnormal foci apart from known left PN

9.3 I-123 MIBG/I-131 MIBG

Clinical Use Localization and treatment of tumors that arise in neuroectodermal tissues (pheochromocytomas, neuroblastomas, carcinoid tumors, medullary thyroid tumors, paragangliomas, and chemodectomas).

I-131 t_{phys} 8 days. *Decays* β- (606 KeV), <u>gamma photon</u> E 364 keV. *Production* fission of U-235.

I-123 Cyclotron-produced t_{phys}: 13.3 h. *Emits*: gamma photons 159 keV.

MIBG Metaiodobenzylguanidine (Iobenguane) norepinephrine analog.
   I-123 MIBG: Used for localization and pre/post-I-131 treatment evaluation.
   I-131 MIBG: Mainly used for neuroendocrine tumor ablation (high dose), can be used for localization (low dose).
   Mechanism: Norepinephrine analog. Taken up in cytoplasmic synaptic vesicles by the presynaptic adrenergic axons via type I, energy-dependent, active amine transport mechanism.

Protocol

Patient preparation:
   <u>Medication to be stopped prior to exam.</u>
   Tricyclic antidepressants and related drugs – avoid for 6 weeks.
   Antihypertensives (Ca channel blocker, labetalol, reserpine) – avoid 2 weeks.
   Sympathetic amines (pseudoephedrine, phenylpropanolamine, phenylephrine, ephedrine) – avoid 2 weeks.
   Cocaine – avoid 2 weeks.
   <u>Thyroid block</u>
   I-123 MIBG Lugol's solution – 5 drops orally 1 h before radiotracer injection, 5 drops same day night and next morning.
   I-131 MIBG (treatment) 5 drops every day starting 3 days prior the exam and 2 weeks after. (SSKI or potassium perchlorate can also be used). *CAUTION: Giving K perchlorate for more than a few days can cause aplastic anemia.*

Dose I-123 MIBG 5–10 mCi/I-131 MIBG 0.5 mCi. I-131 MIBG 200–400 mCi (treatment as inpatient under radiation safety guidelines).
   Prior to treatment with I-131 – inject 1 mCi of Tc-99m pertechnetate/DTPA IV, for line patency.

Image I-123 MIBG – 24 h images. I-131: 7–14 days posttreatment.

Critical Organ I *-123 MIBG* Bladder *I-131 MIBG* liver.

Distribution Adrenal medulla, heart, salivary glands, and spleen (rich adrenergic innervations). 20 % GI tract (free iodine).

Clearance Renal: about 40–50 % within 24 h, 70–90 % within 4 days.

Distribution and Clearance

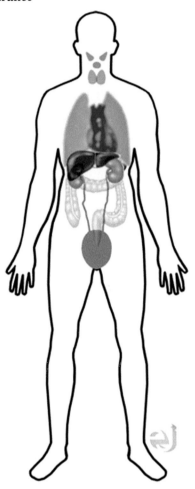

Distribution Adrenal medulla, heart, salivary glands, lung, spleen, and liver (rich adrenergic innervations), 20 % GI tract (free iodine).
Clearance Renal; about 40–50 % within 24 h, 70–90 % within 4 days.

Distribution and Clearance

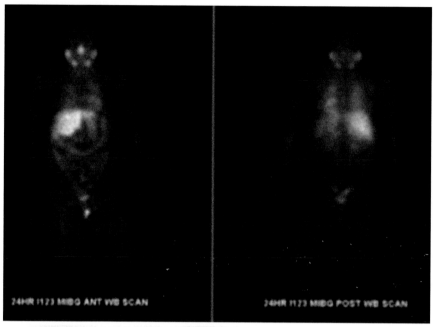

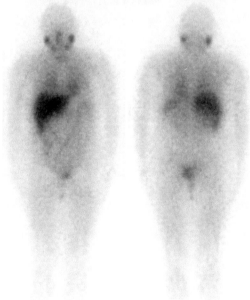

Distribution Adrenal medulla, heart, salivary glands, spleen, and<<< liver (rich adrenergic innervations), 20 % GI tract (free iodine).
Clearance Renal; about 40–50 % within 24 h, 70–90 % within 4 days.

Abnormal Distribution

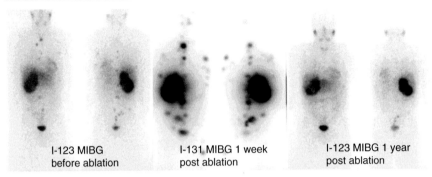

I-123 MIBG
before ablation

I-131 MIBG 1 week
post ablation

I-123 MIBG 1 year
post ablation

Metastatic pheochromocytoma

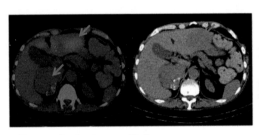

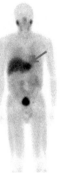

Neuroendocrine tumor with liver
metastasis

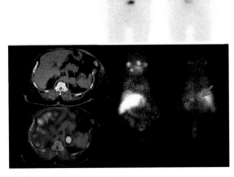

Pheochromocytoma

10   Kidneys

10.1 Renal Scintigraphy

Indication Evaluation of renal function and obstruction (mechanical or functional).

Tc-99m Generator produced in the form of Tc-99m pertechnetate (TcO_4^{1-}) (+7 valence) from Mo-99. t_{phys} 6 h. *Emits*: gamma 140 keV (89 %).

Pharmaceuticals Dimercaptosuccinic acid (DMSA), glucoheptonate (GH), diethylenetriaminepentaacetic acid (DTPA), mercaptoacetyltriglycine (MAG3).

Mechanism and Distribution

Radiopharmaceuticals	Mechanism	Advantages	Use (approximately)
Tc-99m-MAG3	EF-40 %. Tubular secretion	Great ROI/BKG	>75 % use
Tc-99m-DTPA	EF-20 %. Glomeruli filtration (GF)	Good quality – when function is good	20 % use
Tc-99m-DMSA	Cortical binding 40 %	Split function/ pyelonephritis	2 % mainly pediatric use
Tc-99m-GH	10–15 % cortical, 85–90 % GF	Split function/ pyelonephritis	1 % (as an alternative to DMSA)

EF extraction fraction

   Tc-99m DMSA: 40 % will be retained in the renal tubules within 1 h. DMSA is initially bound to α1-microglobulin → Tc-99m DMSA α1-microglobulin complex → filtered by the glomerulus → accumulates in the kidneys via megalin/tubulin-mediated endocytosis from the glomerular filtrate (Andrew 2014; Weyer et al. 2013)

   Tc-99m GH: Good alternative to DMSA if not available. Predominantly glomerular filtration agent. Ten to fifteen percent will be retained in the tubules. Use as cortical imaging agent (cannot be used for renogram).

   Tc-99m DTPA: Extraction fraction is 20 %. Purely filtered by the glomerulus. Calculates GFR.

   Tc-99m-MAG3: Highly protein bound. Extraction fraction is 40–50 %. Extraction from the plasma lumen by the organic anion transporter 1 in the basolateral membrane. Transported into the tubular lumen via organic anion transporters on the apical membrane. Small fraction will be cleared via the hepatobiliary system (Weyer et al. 2013; Shikano et al. 2004; Eshima and Taylor 1992; Bubeck et al. 1990).

Suggested Reading

- Andrew T (2014). Taylor; radionuclides in nephrourology, Part 1: radiopharmaceuticals, quality control, and quantitative indices. J Nucl Med 55:608–615
- Bubeck B, Brandau W, Weber E, Kälble T, Parekh N, Georgi P (1990). Pharmacokinetics of technetium-99m-MAG3 in humans. J Nucl Med 31: 1285–1293
- Eshima D, Taylor A Jr. (1992). Technetium-99m (99mTc) mercaptoacetyltriglycine: update on the new 99mTc renal tubular function agent. Semin Nucl Med 22:61–73
- Shikano N, Kanai Y, Kawai K, Ishikawa N, Endou H (2004). Transport of 99mTc-MAG3 via rat renal organic anion transporter 1. J Nucl Med 45:80–85
- Weyer K et al (2013). Renal uptake of 99mTc dimercaptosuccinic acid is dependent on normal proximal tubule receptor-mediated endocytosis. J Nucl Med 54:159–165

Distribution and Clearance

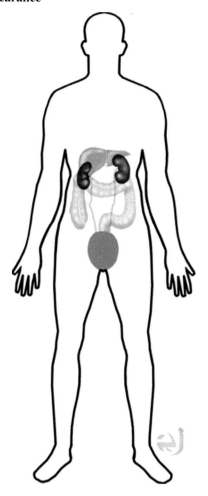

Distribution Highly protein bound. Extraction fraction by the kidney is 40–50 %.
Clearance Secreted by the kidneys. Small fraction will be cleared via hepatobiliary
system.

10.2 Renal Scan Protocols

Cortical Imaging *Radiopharmaceuticals*: Tc-99m DMSA (more commonly used), Tc-99m GH (rarely used).

Dose: Pediatrics – 50 µCi/kg (minimum dose of 600 µCi) Adult: 5 mCi *Imaging protocol*: Posterior images with LEAP collimator for differential split calculation. Continue with right and left pinhole for detailed cortical images (pediatrics, larger images – better spatial resolution)

Renal Scintigraphy *Radiopharmaceuticals*: Tc-99m MAG3 (more commonly used) or Tc-99m DTPA.

Dose: 10 mCi of Tc-99m MAG3 or Tc- 99m DTPA.

Imaging protocol: Hydration – Arrive well hydrated (drink two large glasses of water just before arrival), void immediately before the study. Image – Supine posterior. Two-phase protocol: *Base line image – flow* 1–2 s/image for 1 min → followed by *dynamic images* for 20–30 min (10- to 20-s frames and are usually displayed at 1- or 2-min intervals). *Diuresis phase* – If obstruction is suspected, repeat above after giving diuresis. One-phase protocol: (F = furosemide) *F = −15, +10, +20* : Give furosemide (Lasix) 15 min prior to or 10, 20 min after the injection of tracer, respectively. *F = 0* Give Lasix with the injection of the tracer. *Lasix dose*: creatinine (mg/Dl): furosemide (mg) → 1.0:20, 1.5:40, 2.0:60, >2.5:80. Conclusion of the study: postvoid images (normal is less than 30 % bladder residual)

Quantitation (Time-Activity Curve)

Measurements of function: <u>MAG3 clearance</u> – normal should be within expected range for age (240–340 ml/min) — software analysis. Decreases 1 % every year. <u>Relative uptake</u> ROI over each kidney 2–3 min postinjection, normal is 42–58 %, <u>time to peak or Tmax</u> normal < 5 min, <u>20 min counts/Tmax or 20 to max ratio</u> normal is approx. 0.34

   Measurements of obstruction: $T_{\frac{1}{2}}$ normal is <10 min, obstructed >20 min, 10–20 min – equivocal

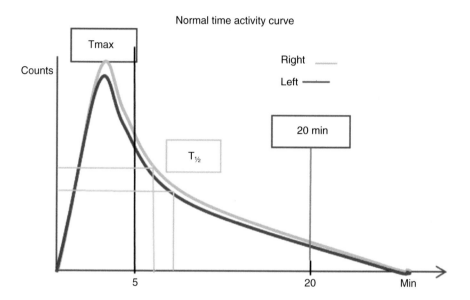

Suggested Reading

- Hunsche A, Press H, Taylor A (2004). Increasing the dose of furosemide in patients with azotemia and suspected obstruction. Clin Nucl Med 29:149–153
- Taylor AT, Shenvi N, Folks RD, Garcia EV, Savir-Baruch B, Manatunga A (2013). Reference values for renal size obtained from MAG3 scintigraphy. Clin Nucl Med 38:13–17

10.3 Renal Scans Pitfalls

Acute Tubular Necrosis (ATN) Normal perfusion. No secretion of tracer from the cortex to the collecting system. Improves with time. More common after nonliving donor transplant.

Rejection Perfusion is the key → decreases with time. Biopsy is gold standard for diagnosis. Differentiation between acute or chronic is usually determined clinically.

High-Grade Obstruction Looks like ATN. Usually history of ureteroureterostomy. 2 h delay images will demonstrate tracer washout until the obstruction point.

Ileal Conduit/Indiana Pouch Reflux can mimic obstruction – place a Foley.

Nephrostomy Tube Clamp only when there is a question of obstruction via the ureters.

Dehydration Falsely increases 20/max ratio value due to dehydration.

Region of Interest (ROI) Determine the renogram time-activity curve. Should be assessed regularly.

Hydronephrosis Recommended to separate the renal cortex ROI from the whole kidney for measurements of cortical function (Tmax and 20/max ratio).

Pelvic Kidney Use geometric mean with anterior and posterior images to account for tissue attenuation when calculating split function.

$$\text{Geometric Mean} = \sqrt{\text{Anterior cts} \times \text{Posterior cts}}$$

Gravity Always look at postvoid images. Gravity will increase tracer washout.

Tc-MAG3 Normal Tracer Distribution

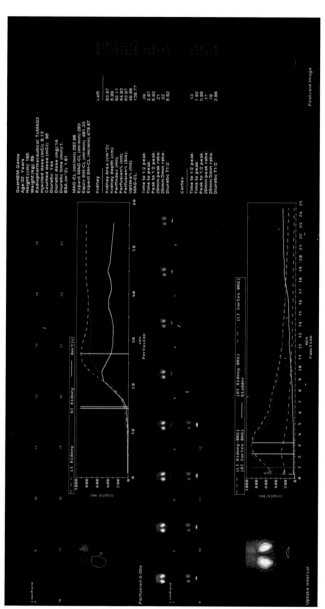

Quantitation

Measurements of function: <u>MAG3 clearance</u> – normal should be within expected range for age (240–340 ml/min) – software analysis. Decreases 1 % every year, <u>relative uptake</u>: ROI over each kidney 2–3 min postinjection, normal is 42–58 %, <u>Time to peak or T_{max}</u>: Normal <5 min, <u>20 min counts/T_{max}</u> or 20 to max ratio normal is approx. 0.34.

Measurements of obstruction: <u>$T_{1/2}$</u> normal is <10 min, obstructed >20 min, 10–20 min – equivocal

Tc-MAG3 Normal Tracer Distribution

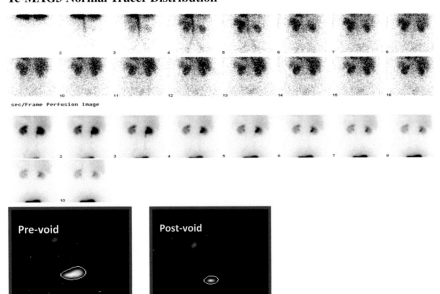

sec/Frame Perfusion Image

Pre-void

Post-void

Tc-MAG3 Abnormal Scans

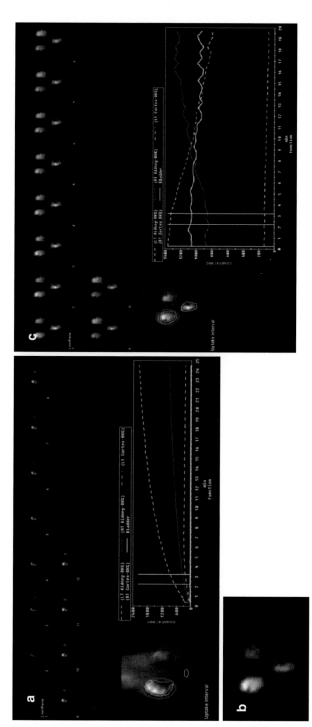

Patient with ileal conduit. (a) Pre-Lasix images: bilateral delay tracer renal uptake. (b) Post void images: Right kidney demonstrates near washout. (c) Post-Lasix images in the supine position demonstrate reflux to the right kidney.

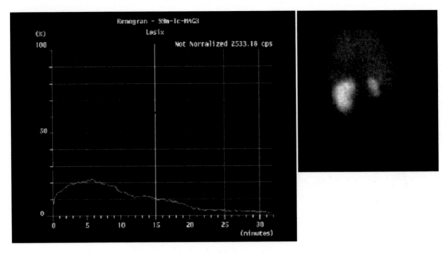

Patient with poor right renal function. Split function is 80:20 %, left:right % kidney

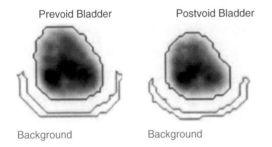

Patient with abnormal bladder emptying. % residual: 72 % (Normal is <30 %)

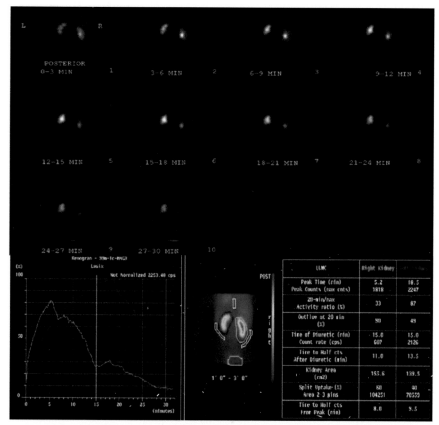

Left hydronephrosis. Evaluation of obstruction. Left kidney dynamic Pre-Lasix images demonstrate delay tracer uptake with T_{max} of 10.5 min (normal value <5 min) and tracer retention within the left renal pelvis. Post -Lasix images demonstrate rapid washout with $T_{1/2}$ of 9.5 (normal is below 10 min).

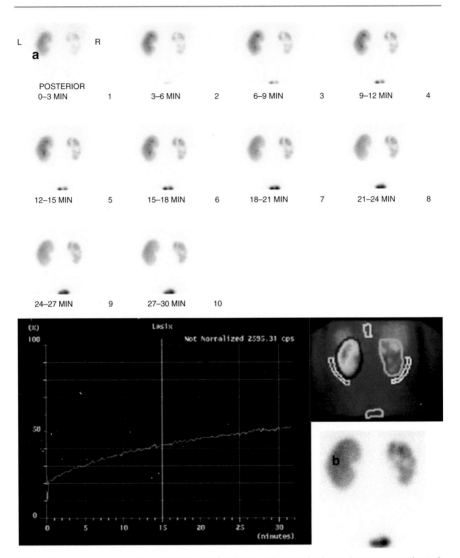

Bilateral functional obstruction. Patient with Cr of 1.2 and normal urine volume was evaluated for removal of right ureteral stent. (a) Dynamic Pre and Post-Lasix images and activity curve demonstrate poor right kidney function (split function is 72:28 % L:R). As well, bilateral delayed tracer uptake with no secretion. (b) Post void images: Significant tracer residual with in the cortex bilaterally.

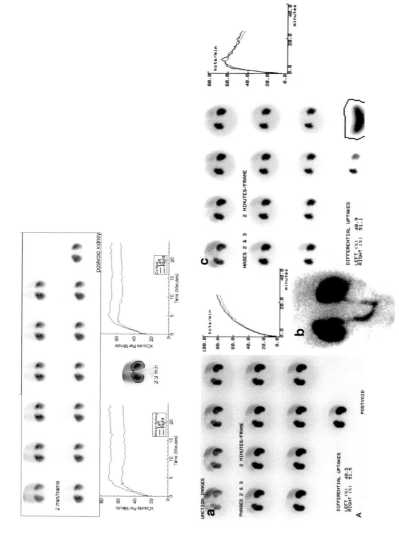

Upper: Acute tubular necrosis (ATN). Normal uptake. Persistent nephrogram. Lower: (a) High grade obstruction: with persistent nephrogram. (b) 2-h delay images demonstrate no washout beyond point of obstruction. Patient had ureteroureterostomy. (c) After correction of anastomosis stricture, repeat study demonstrates resolution of obstruction.

10.4 Renovascular Hypertension (Angiotensin-Converting Enzyme [ACE] Inhibition Renography)

Indication   Assess for hypertension secondary to renal artery stenosis.

Radiopharmaceuticals   Tc-99m MAG3 (more commonly used) or Tc-99m DTPA.

Dose   *Baseline:* 1 mCi of Tc-99m MAG3 or Tc-99m DTPA followed by 10 mCi after ACE inhibitor (ACEI) challenge.
ACE inhibitors: captopril: 25–50 mg PO, enalaprilat: 40 µg/kg IV over 3–5 min, maximum dose of 2.5 mg.

Mechanism

Renin-angiotensin system:
1. Renin – peptide hormone secreted from the juxtaglomerular cells of the afferent arteriole due to renal hypoperfusion, decreased distal chloride delivery to the macula densa and increased sympathetic activity.
2. Angiotensinogen: synthesizes and secretes from the liver.
3. Angiotensin $\overset{\text{Renin}}{\longrightarrow}$ Angiotensin I (cleaved).
4. Angiotensin I $\overset{\text{ACE}}{\longrightarrow}$ angiotensin II.
5. Systemic vasoconstrictor and renal *efferent* arterial vasoconstriction → maintain GFR.

ACE inhibitor

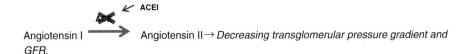

Angiotensin I   ⟶   Angiotensin II → *Decreasing transglomerular pressure gradient and GFR.*

Protocol

Preparation Discontinuing ACE inhibitors 2–3 days for captopril and 5–7 days for long-acting ACEI. Ingest 7 ml water/kg 30–60 min prior to exam.

One-day protocol

1. *Obtain baseline images*: Inject 1 mCi of tracer followed by no Lasix renal scintigraphy protocol. Some protocols suggest the use of 20 mg Lasix at 2 minutes of each study.
2. *ACE inhibitor challenge*: Crushed captopril into 150–250 ml of water and give it PO. Wait for 60 min prior to tracer administration or give IV form (enalaprilat) and wait for 15 min. Repeat renal scintigraphy protocol with 10 mCi of Tc-99m MAG3 or Tc-99m DTPA.

Two-days protocol
ACEI phase should be performed first.

1. If time-activity curve is normal → study is concluded.
2. If abnormal → bring patient back the day after and repeat the study for "baseline" (no ACE inhibitor) images.

Interpretation   Look for changes in the time activity curve between base-line and post ACE inhibitor challenge phases:

- **Type 0** : Normal
- **Type 1** : T_{max} of >5 min and 20-min/maximum count ratio of > 0.3
- **Type 2** : More exaggerated delays in time to peak and in parenchymal washout
- **Type 3** : Progressive parenchymal accumulation (no washout detected)
- **Type 4** : Renal failure pattern but with measurable renal uptake
- **Type 5** : Renal failure pattern representing blood background activity only

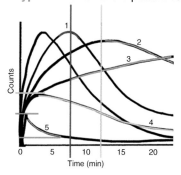

Suggested Reading
Taylor et al (2003). Society of Nuclear Medicine Procedure Guideline for Diagnosis of Renovascular Hypertension SNMMI 6

10.5 Renovascular Hypertension, ACE Inhibition Renography: Abnormal Pattern

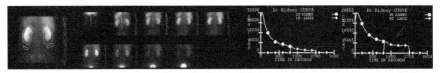

Baseline images with normal bilateral renal function.

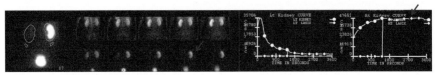

MAG3 administered 1.5 h post-captopril

Right kidney function significantly decreased. No tracer secretion to the renal pelvis. Positive for right renal artery stenosis.

11 Bladder

11.1 Tc-99m Sulfur Colloid-Voiding Cystourethrogram (VCUG)

Indication Evaluation for ureteral reflux.

Tc-99m Generator produced in the form of Tc-99m pertechnetate (TcO_4^{1-}) (+7 valence) from Mo-99. t_{phys} 6 h. *Emits* gamma 140 keV (89 %).

Sulfur Colloid Particle size of 0.1–2.0 μm.

Tc-99m SC Preparation kit *does not include stannous* to bind TcO_4^{1-} with SC – the *only* Tc-99m tracer that does not require stannous ion.

Mechanism of Action Via Foley catheter: Tc-99m SC particles mixed with normal saline will occupy the bladder space.

Protocol Tc-99m sulfur colloid will be injected in a retrograde fashion via a Foley Catheter → followed by administration of normal saline into the bladder by gravity – until maximum tolerance is achieved or formulated volume is given. Bladder capacity volume in children = (age in years + 2) × 30 cc. Images will be obtained every constant volume in the posterior position. Also, static images of full bladder, voiding, and postvoid phases. Bladder region of interest will be calculated using residual volume (RV) formula.

$$RV(mL) = \frac{\text{Voided volume}(mL) \times \text{Post} - \text{void bladder counts}(ROI)}{\text{Initial bladder counts}(ROI) - \text{Post} - \text{void bladder counts}(ROI)}$$

Dose Adult: 1–2 mCi; Child: (5 years old) 0.5–1.0 mCi.

Target Organ Bladder.

Abnormal Distribution Reflux of the tracer into:

Grade 1 – A nondilated ureter.
Grade 2 – A nondilated calyces.
Grade 3 – Mildly dilated ureter and renal pelvis.
Grade 4 – Moderately dilated renal calyces with ureteral tuberosity.
Grade 5 – Severe dilatation of the renal pelvis, calyces, ureteral tuberosity, and loss of papillary impressions.

Suggested Reading
- Society of Nuclear Medicine Procedure Guideline for Radionuclide Cystography

Distribution Patterns

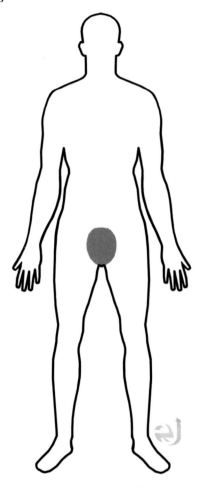

Clearance Via Foley Urinating

Normal Versus Abnormal Distribution

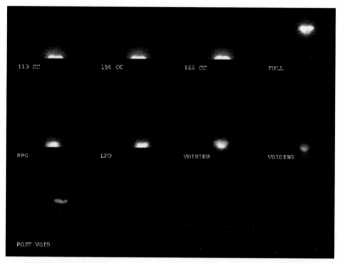

Normal – No reflux

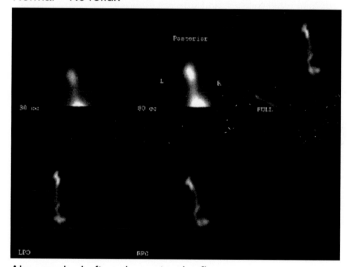

Abnormal – Left vesicoureteral reflux

12 Prostate

12.1 ProstaScint: Indium-111 Capromab Pendetide

Indications Newly diagnosed patients with Biopsy (+) prostate cancer (PCA), after standard imaging, with high risk for metastases. Post-prostatectomy patients with rising PSA and negative standard images associated with high clinical suspicion for metastatic disease.

Indium-111 Cyclotron produced from cadmium (Cd-112) target. t_{phys} 2.83 days (67 h). *Emits* gamma 173 (89 %) and 247 (94 %) keV.

ProstaScint Murine monoclonal Ab (CYT 356) conjugated to the chelator (GYT-DTA) → intact murine immunoglobulin.

Mechanism ProstaScint antibody directed against *prostate-specific membrane antigen* (PSMA) – type II membrane protein, located in the cytoplasmic domain (intracellular) of prostate cell. Other locations of low PSMA expression: Small intestine, proximal renal tubules, and salivary glands.

Protocol

Patient preparation (1) Murine monoclonal antibodies (any subtype) can induce HAMA elevation leading to immune reaction. Therefore, HAMA level should be checked prior to injection (2) Bowel prep 2 days prior to injection.

Dose 5 mCi, IV injection.

Imaging 3–5 days postinjection (Avg 96 h) whole-body planar images + SPECT/CT.

Critical Organ Liver.

Interpretation Only by experts, due to high blood pool activity, special attention to anatomical localization of LN is needed. Positive lesions: intensity is > blood pool.

Distribution *Early* blood pool. *96 h*, Liver spleen, bone marrow, and blood pool.

Clearance Kidney >>> bowel.

Distribution and Clearance

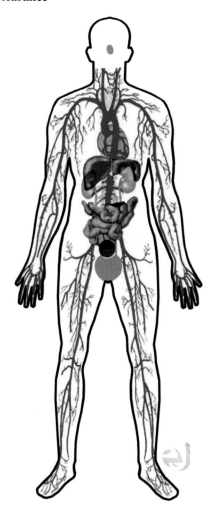

Distribution Blood pool activity up to 96 h. Liver, spleen, bone marrow, and blood pool.
Clearance Kidney >>> bowel.

Distribution and Clearance

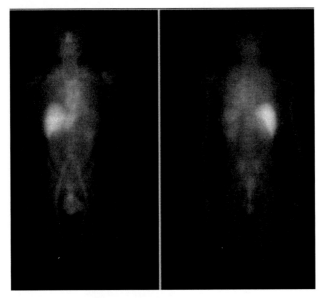

Planar images. Whole body distribution

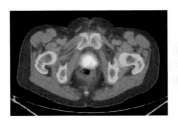

SPECT/CT. Prostate gland uptake

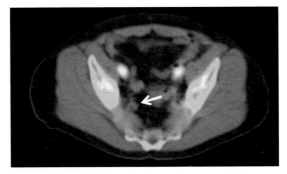

SPECT/CT. Right common iliac Lymph
node suspicious for recurrence with no
increase uptake

Part 3: Clinical Nuclear Medicine – Whole-Body Scans

Contents

© Springer International Publishing Switzerland 2017
B. Savir-Baruch, B.J. Barron, *RadTool Nuclear Medicine Flash Facts*,
DOI 10.1007/978-3-319-24636-9_3

1　Infections and Inflammations

1.1　Gallium-67 Citrate Scan

Indications
1. Lymphoma (HD>NHL).
2. Solid tumors (lung, melanoma, HCC (hepatoma), sarcoma, testicular tumor, head and neck cancers, neuroblastoma.
3. Infections and inflammations (vertebral osteomyelitis – better than In-111 WBC), fever of unknown origin (FUO), fungal infections, granulomatous diseases, and sarcoidosis.

Ga-67 Citrate t_{phys} 78 h. Cyclotron produced, decays by electron capture (EC). *Emits* gamma radiation 93 (37 %), 185 (20 %), 300 (17 %), and 395 (5 %). Known as "90, 190, 290, and 390."

Mechanisms of Action Iron analog. Will not cross the BBB (blood brain barrier). *Infections:* Ga-67 binding affinity – lactoferrin >>siderophores>transferrin. Leukocytes will secrete lactoferrin (lactoferrin mechanism), and bacteria will secrete siderophores. Ga-67 – bound to transferrin → transported via blood stream to infection site → attached to lactoferrin >>>and siderophores.

Solid tumors: Transmembrane transferrin receptor (CD71) on tumor cells via endocytosis (transferrin mechanism), then attached to lysosomal proteins.

Lymphomas: Transferrin and lactoferrin mechanism.

Protocol Bowel prep. optional → IV injection → 48–72 h, whole body scan + SPECT/CT of the chest/abdomen at 48 or 72 h. Can wait up to 7–10 days to image (e.g., differentiate intra-abdominal infection from normal bowel clearance).

Dose Infection (5 mCi), tumor imaging (10 mCi).

Imaging Collimator – medium energy parallel, 20 % windows at 93, 185, and 300 KeV or 20 % windows at 93 and 185 KeV. Whole-body planar anterior posterior images followed by SPECT/CT of region of interest (chest/abdomen and pelvis).

Critical Organ Colon.

Distribution Blood pool (plasma protein bound %) – 24 h, 20 %; 48 h, 10 %; and 72 h, 5 %.

Infection site/tumor uptake at 12–24 h.

Liver > bone marrow >>> colon (variable uptake), lacrimal gland, nasopharyngeal, breasts (cycle variant), testes, lung, thymus (peds), spleen, kidneys.

Clearance *First 24 h* – 25 % clearance by kidneys. *> 24 h* – bowel>>kidneys (kidney uptake is abnormal at 48 h).

Variations
A. Chemotherapy decreases liver activity significantly.
B. Scrotal uptake may be normal.
C. Imaging quality: Poor due to "downscatter" from high-energy photons not being imaged.
D. Weak bone agent. Discordance with bone scan – infection is less likely.
E. Sarcoidosis involving the salivary glands will demonstrate intense Ga67 uptake also known as the "panda sign".

Distribution and Clearance

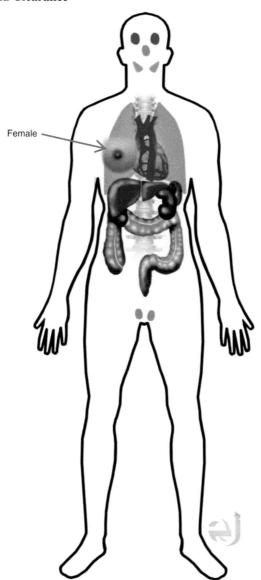

Distribution

Blood pool (plasma protein bound %) – 24 h, 20 %; 48 h, 10 %; and 72 h, 5 %. Infection site/tumor uptake at 12–24 h.

Liver > bone marrow >>> colon (variable uptake), lacrimal gland, nasopharyngeal, breasts (cycle variant), testes, lung, thymus (peds), spleen, kidneys.

Clearance (1) First 24 h – 25 % clearance by kidneys. (2) ≥ 24 h – bowel>>kidneys. (3) 48 h – 75 % tracer in body.

Normal Distribution

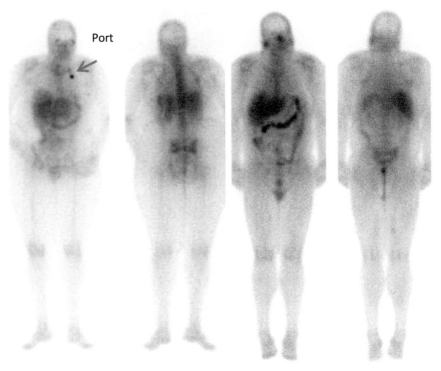

Port

Distribution

Blood pool (plasma protein bound %) – 24 h, 20 %; 48 h, 10 %; and 72 h, 5 %. Infection site/tumor uptake at 12–24 h.

Liver > bone marrow >> > colon (variable uptake), lacrimal gland, nasopharyngeal, breasts (cycle variant), testes, lung, thymus (peds), spleen, kidneys.

Clearance (1) First 24 h – 25 % clearance by kidneys. (2) ≥ 24 h – bowel>>kidneys. (3) 48 h – 75 % tracer in body.

Abnormal Distribution

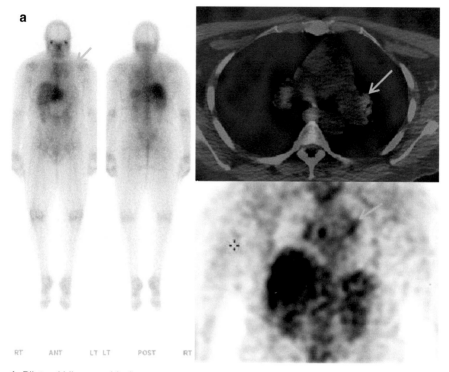

A. Bilateral hilar sarcoidosis

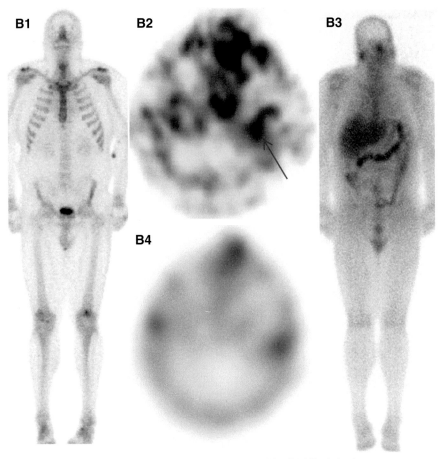

B. Bone scan suspicious for left petrous bone osteomyelitis. *B1.* Whole body
   images – normal. *B2.* SPECT images demonstrate abnormality. *B3.* Ga-67 Planar and
   B4. SPECT images are negative. Acute infection was ruled out.
   Diagnosis: Chronic inflammation.

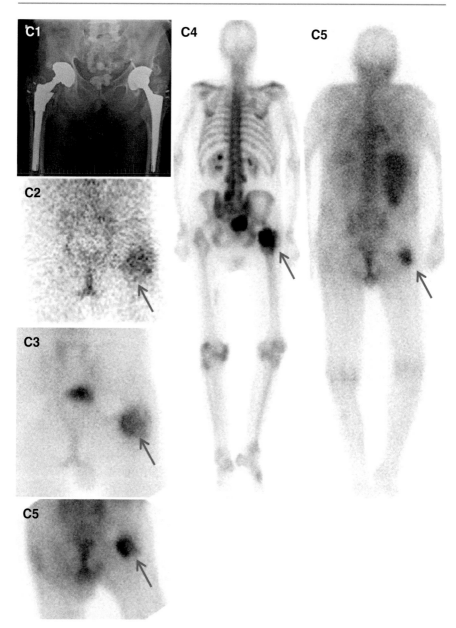

C. 1. Patient with bilateral hip replacement hardware. Three Phase Bone Scan in the posterior
   views (2. Flow 3. Blood pool 4. Delay) demonstrate abnormal right hip tracer uptake,
   suspicious for osteomyelitis/infected hardware. 5. 24 h Ga-67 scan confirms the diagnosis.

1.2   Indium-111 Oxine-Labeled WBC

Indications Infection localization.

Indium-111 Cyclotron produced from cadmium (Cd-112) target. t_{phys} 2.83 days (67 h). *Emits* gamma 173 (89 %) and 247 (94 %) KeV.

Oxine (8-Hydroxyquinoline) Lipid-soluble complex (chelate).

Risks Auger electrons of 0.6–25.4 keV → damage labeled cells → lymphocytes are more radiosensitive and longer lived → mutagenic and oncogenic effects. Therefore, this exam is only for adults.

Mechanism Labeled WBC will be reinjected into the patient, and one will follow its physiological distribution (infection localization).

Protocol

Serum WBC should be >>5,000/mm³ (min value of 3,000/mm³).

Draw 30–50 ml.

Isolate leukocytes: Sedimentation and centrifugation (WBC in the bottom).

Radiolabel with ~1,000 μCi of In-111 oxine to prepare a 500 μCi dose for injection.

Inject by two healthcare professionals (blood product protocol).

Image 24 h planar images (whole body if site of infection is unknown) +/- SPECT/ CT as indicated. For inflammatory bowel disease (IBD) image at 4 h following by 24 h. Tc99m labeled WBC is more sensitive for IBD detection with 30 min – 2 h post injection images.

Critical Organ Spleen.

Distribution

Initial – blood pool, lungs, liver, and spleen. Lung activity secondary to margination of WBCs.

4 h lung activity and blood pool normally decrease, although not always completely.

24 h spleen, followed by the liver and then the bone marrow (BM).

Variant GI activity often secondary to sinus drainage. Poor labeling technique – persistent blood pool at 24 h indicates a high percentage of labeled erythrocytes or platelets.

Clearance Clears from the blood circulation with t_{eff}=7.5 h; localizes in WBC pool organs (spleen, liver, and BM).

False Negative Encapsulated nonpyogenic abscess; vertebral osteomyelitis; chronic low-grade infection; parasitic; mycobacterial or fungal infections; intrahepatic, perihepatic, or splenic infection; hyperglycemia; steroids.

False Positive Gastrointestinal bleeding; pseudoaneurysm; healing fracture; soft tissue tumor; swallowed leukocytes; oropharyngeal, esophageal, or lung disease; surgical wounds, stomas, or catheter sites; hematomas; tumors; accessory spleens; renal transplant.

Distribution and Clearance

4 h   24 h

Distribution *4 h* – spleen > liver >>> bone marrow > lung. Activity and blood pool normally decrease, although not always completely

24 h – spleen > liver >>>> bone marrow

Clearance Clears from the blood circulation with $t_{eff} = 7.5$ h; localizes in WBC pool organs (spleen, liver, and BM).

Distribution and Clearance

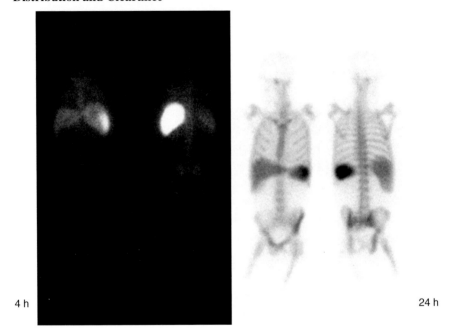

4 h   24 h

Distribution *4 h* – spleen > liver >>> bone marrow > lung. Activity and blood pool normally decrease, although not always completely.

  24 h – spleen > liver >>>> bone marrow.

Clearance Clears from the blood circulation in 7.5 h (t_{eff}) to WBC pool organs (spleen, liver, and BM).

Abnormal Distribution

Flow	Blood pool	Delay	In-111WBC

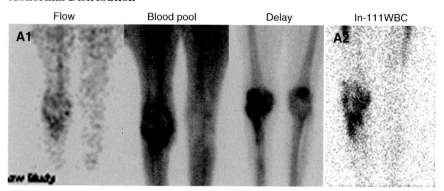

A.1 Three-phase bone scan and In-111 WBC scans (A.2) positive for septic right knee joint.

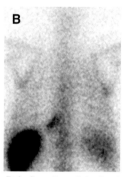

B. Left costovertebral osteomyelitis.

1.3 Tc-99m WBC: Tc-99m Labeled with Hexamethylpropyleneamine Oxime (HMPAO)

Indications *Infection.*

Tc-99m Generator produced in the form of Tc-99m pertechnetate (TcO$_4^{1-}$) from Mo-99. t_{phys} 6 h. *Emits* gamma 140 KeV (89 %).

Mechanism *WBC tagged:* Labeled WBC will be reinjected into the patient and will follow its physiological distribution (infection localization).

Dose 20 mCi.

Protocol

Patient prep. Wound dressing change.

Labeling: 50 ml autologous blood → WBC separation → prepare 20 mCi dose of Tc-99m WBC → reinjection.

Image.

Intra-abdominal /inflammatory bowel disease: Image at 30 min up to 2 h. Commonly done at 2 h postinjection. 24 h images will be obtained as needed (usually if early images are negative).

Osteomyelitis: Image at 4 h followed by 24 h delayed images as needed.

Critical Organ Spleen.

Distribution Spleen > liver >> bowel, bone marrow, kidney, gallbladder, some lung.

Clearance Renal > hepatobiliary.

Distribution and Clearance

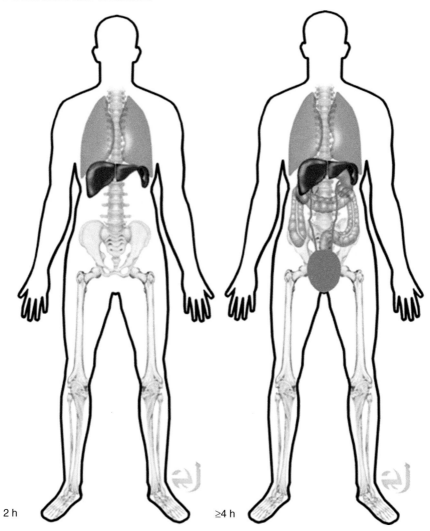

2 h   ≥4 h

Distribution Spleen > liver >> bowel, bone marrow, kidney, gallbladder, some lung.
Clearance Renal > hepatobiliary.

Distribution and Clearance

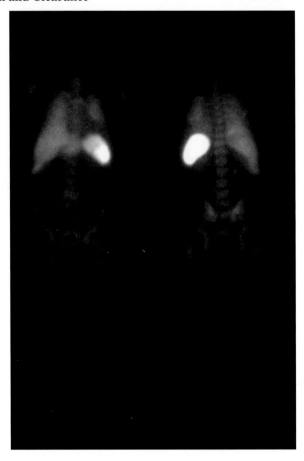

Distribution Spleen > liver >> bowel, bone marrow, kidney, gallbladder, some lung.
Clearance *Tagged WBC:* Renal > hepatobiliary.

Abnormal Distribution

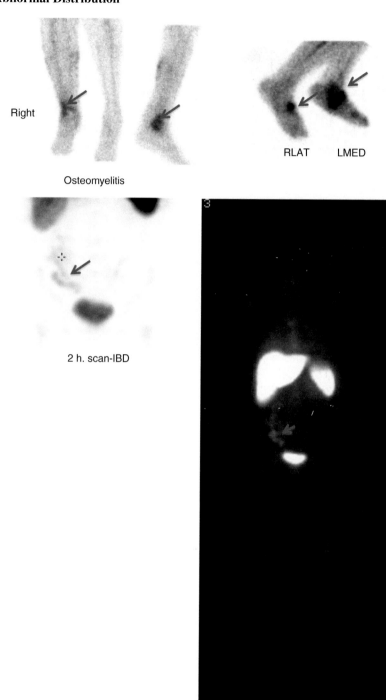

Right

Osteomyelitis

RLAT   LMED

2 h. scan-IBD

Tc-99m WBC Versus In-111 WBC

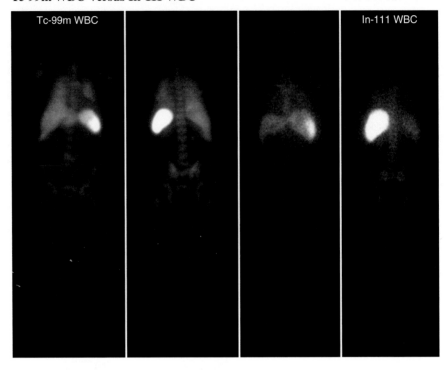

2   Skeleton

2.1   Tc-99m Methylene Diphosphonate (Tc-99m MDP)

Tc-99m Generator produced in the form of Tc-99m pertechnetate (TcO_4^{1-}) (+7 valence) from Mo-99. t_{phys} 6 h. *Emits* gamma 140 KeV (89 %).

MDP Diphosphonates are bisphosphonates = polyphosphates and are chemically analogous to pyrophosphate. High affinity for hydroxyapatite at the *bone surface (also binds to Fe, amyloid, and collagen).*

Mechanism of Action *Osseous uptake:* Diphosphonate will be most effective during active bone remodeling and high amorphous calcium phosphate matrix. It will be adsorbed on the surface of the hydroxyapatite crystals to inhibit osteoclasts.

Extraosseous uptake: Diphosphonate uptake occurs in damaged tissue due to calcium deposition (necrosis, infarct, hypercalcemia).

Protocol

Prep.: (1) Hydration. (2) Void prior and after injection (decrease radiation to bladder).

Dose: 20–25 mCi.

Image:

Whole-body (WB) bone scan: 2.5–4 h postinjection, AP whole-body images followed by static images of region of interest (ROI) and SPECT/CT as indicated.

Three-phase bone scan concept: The two first phases will measure areas of hyperemia due to vasodilatation secondary to active inflammatory cascades. The last phase will demonstrate level of increased bone turnover. Image ROI only (WB if ROI is unknown).

  Blood flow: Dynamic 2–5 s images for 60 s after injection.

  Blood pool: Static images at 5–10 min postinjection for 5 min or 300 K counts.

  Delayed images: At 4 h followed by WB images. May do fourth phase at 24 h if
    bone to soft tissue ratio is low (e.g., diabetic foot with suspected osteomyelitis – no sufficient soft tissue clearance due to poor blood flow).

Distribution Uptake to the bone will be rapid, and peak of the bone to background will be at 6–12 h. Due to the 6 h half-life of Tc-99m, we image at 2–4 h.

Clearance Kidneys (approximately 50 %, 1 h postinjection).

Image Interpretation *Three-phase osteomyelitis;* ↑↑blood flow, pooling, and delayed.

Three-phase prosthesis loosening: normal blood flow → ↑ pooling → ↑ ↑delayed *three phase. Cellulitis* – ↑↑blood flow, ↑↑pooling, and normal delay.

Whole Body Rapid blood pool clearance to the bone. Accumulates primarily in the osteogenic active bone: Joints, cancer, metabolic disease, degenerative disease, fractures, infection, sites of Ca deposition.

Distribution and Clearance

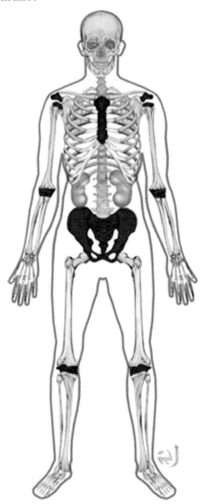

Distribution Uptake to the bone will be rapid, and peak of the bone to background will be at 6–12 h; Tc-99m t_{phys}=6 h → images at 2–4 h.
Clearance Kidneys (approximately 50 %, 1 h postinjection).

Normal Scans

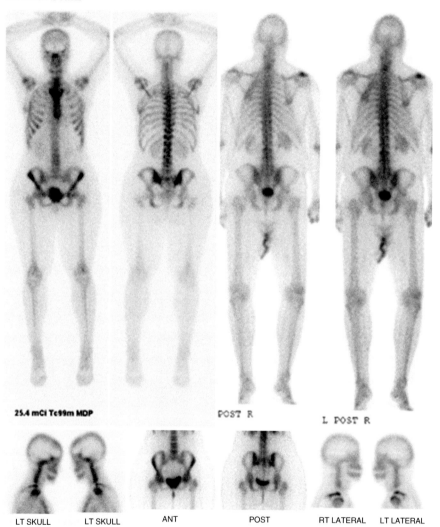

25.4 mCi Tc99m MDP   POST R   L POST R

LT SKULL   LT SKULL   ANT   POST   RT LATERAL   LT LATERAL

Bone Scan (Tc-99m MDP) Common Abnormal Distribution Patterns

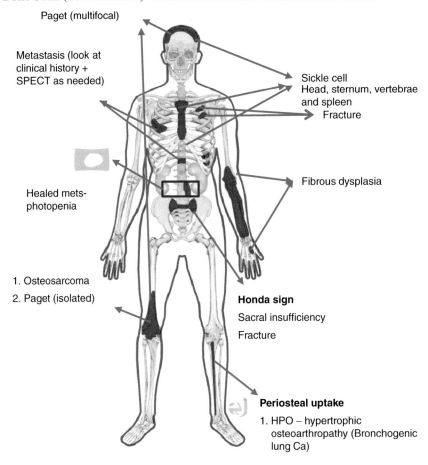

Paget (multifocal)

Metastasis (look at clinical history + SPECT as needed)

Sickle cell
Head, sternum, vertebrae and spleen

Fracture

Fibrous dysplasia

Healed mets-photopenia

1. Osteosarcoma
2. Paget (isolated)

Honda sign

Sacral insufficiency

Fracture

Periosteal uptake

1. HPO – hypertrophic osteoarthropathy (Bronchogenic lung Ca)

2. Shin splints (stress leg soreness)

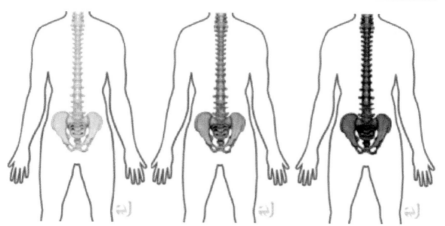

Flare phenomenon: breast cancer diffuse
metastatic interval changes due to healing

Renal osteodystrophy
(diffuse skull uptake)

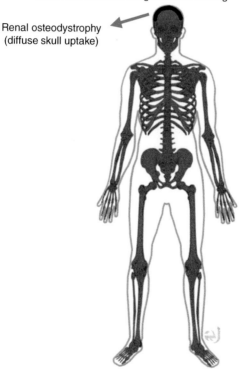

Super scan : No renal clearance
1. Diffuse bony mets (prostate cancer)-
   involved axial and proximal
   appendicular skeleton.
2. Renal osteodystrophy- involved all
   skeleton.

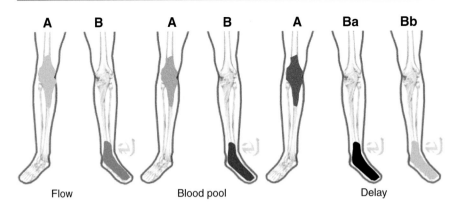

A: Loose prosthesis
Ba: Osteomyelitis
Bb: Cellulitis

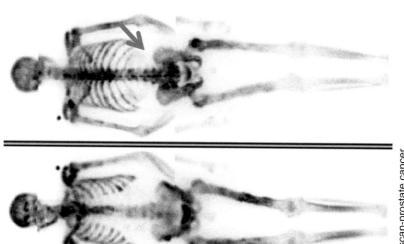

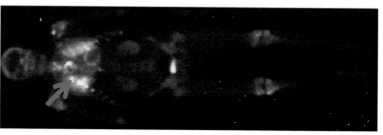

Superscan-prostate cancer.
No renal clearance.

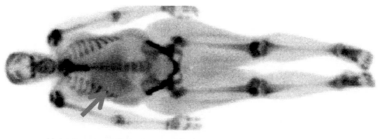

Hypercalcemia

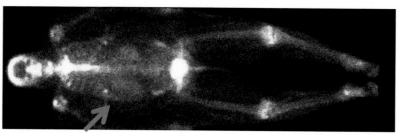

Liver
amyloidosis

Abnormal Distribution

Liver metastasis
breast cancer

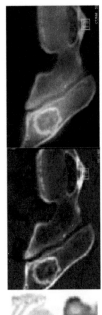

Fibrodysplasia

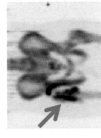

Ectopic bone formation

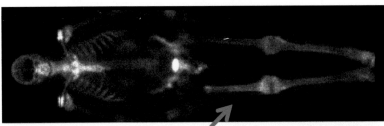

Right femur
osteosarcoma

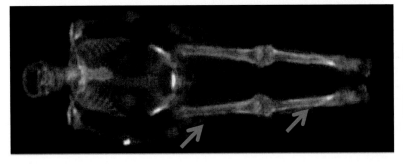

HPO (Lung CA)

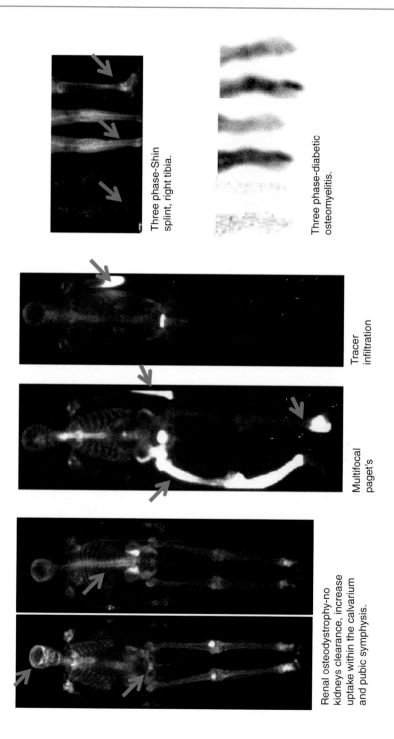

Three phase-Shin splint, right tibia.

Three phase-diabetic osteomyelitis.

Tracer infiltration

Multifocal paget's

Renal osteodystrophy-no kidneys clearance, increase uptake within the calvarium and pubic symphysis.

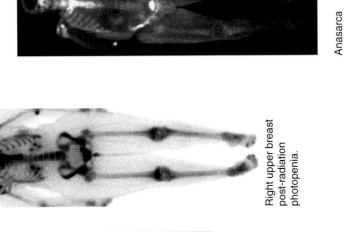

Anasarca

Right upper breast post-radiation photopenia.

Cardiac amyloidosis

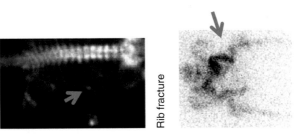

Rib fracture

Cold osteomyelitis

Part 4: FDA-Approved PET/CT Tracers

Contents

© Springer International Publishing Switzerland 2017

B. Savir-Baruch, B.J. Barron, *RadTool Nuclear Medicine Flash Facts*,

DOI 10.1007/978-3-319-24636-9_4

1 FDG

1.1 F-18 Fluorodeoxyglucose (FDG): Positron Emission Tomography (PET/CT)

Clinical Use Oncology, cardiac viability, brain imaging.

18-F Cyclotron produced. t_{phys} 109.8 min. *Decays* positron emission to O-18. 511 KeV photons are emitted (annihilation radiation).

18-FDG Mechanism Glucose metabolism agent. FDG [conversion by hexokinase/glucokinase FDG-6p] → trapped in cell (missing 2' OH groups which are needed for metabolism). After full decay from F-18 to O-18 (heavy oxygen), it will combine with H^+ ion to create 2' OH groups and will be metabolized by glycolysis.

Brain: Scan will demonstrate change in cerebral glucose metabolism associated with foci of epileptic seizures/tumors (please refer to "Flash Facts-Brain Scan").

Cardiac: Normal cells utilize fatty acids as main source of energy; ischemic cells utilize glucose (for more images, please refer to "Flash Fact Cardiac Scans").

Pre-exam sugar load: Increases insulin secretion and decreases protein breakdown to AA → decrease amino acid plasma level → increase glucose uptake by the ischemic myocardial cells.

Oncology: Hexokinase concentration is higher in cancer cells followed by inflammatory cells.

Percentage of Uptake in Myocardium 1–4 %.

Image Protocol

Cardiac viability: (1) Rb-82 rest perfusion protocol. (2) Glucose/insulin load followed by 10 mCi F-18 FDG. (3) 30 min post-FDG injection CT and PET (wait for 60 min for diabetic patients). Nowadays, glucose load is optional.

Oncology/brain: Fasting for 6–8 h (oncology) and 4 h (brain). (1) FDG injection IV. (2) "Cooking" time for 45 min to 1 h to obtain high target to background. (3) CT and PET images.

Imaging PET/CT.

Dose 10–15 mCi.

Critical Organ Bladder.

Distribution Brain >>kidneys, ureters, and bladder>>liver. *Variable*: heart, GI, salivary glands, uterus, ovaries, and testes.

Clearance Kidneys, ureters, and bladder.

Distribution and Clearance

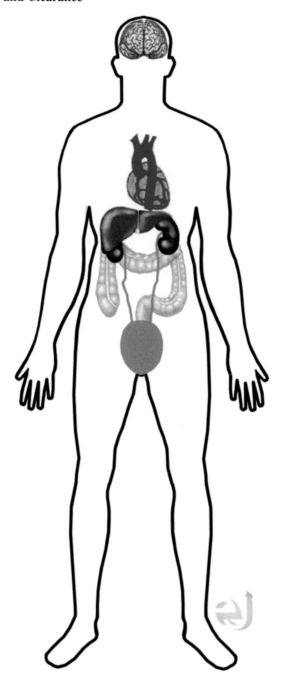

Distribution Brain >>kidneys, ureters, and bladder>>liver. *Variable* – heart, GI, salivary glands, uterus, ovaries, and testes.
Clearance Kidneys, ureters, and bladder.

PET/CT Viability Study

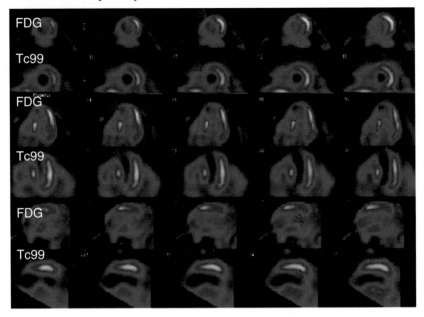

Non-viable LAD distribution
Upper line: FDG PET. Lower line: rest Tc-99m myoview SPECT

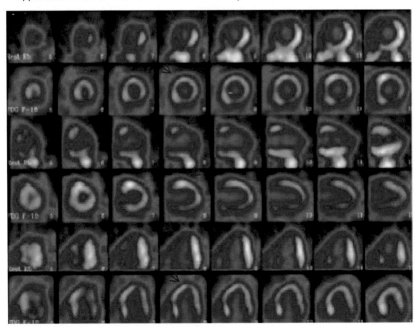

Viable myocardium at the LAD distribution.
Upper line: rest Rb-82 PET. Lower line: FDG PET SPECT

PET/CT Oncology Abnormal Patterpns

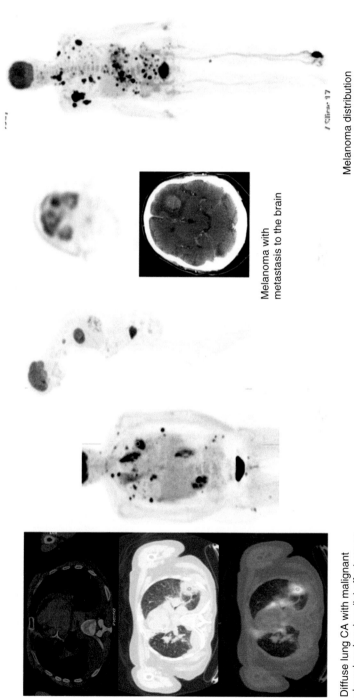

Melanoma distribution pattern presented on maximal intensity projection (MIP) image

Melanoma with metastasis to the brain

Diffuse lung CA with malignant pleural and pericardial effusions as well as subcutaneous nodules

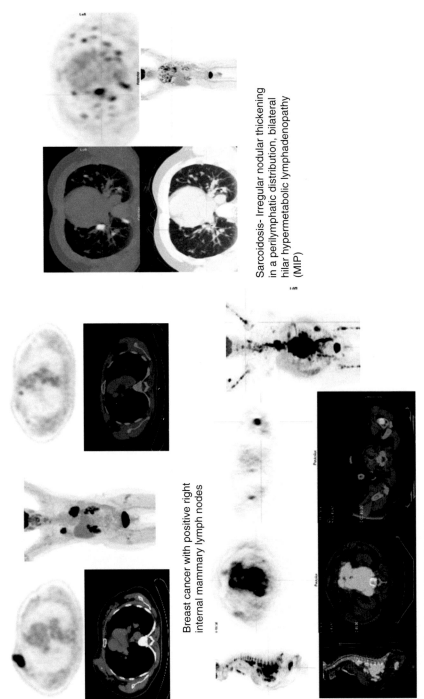

Sarcoidosis- Irregular nodular thickening in a perilymphatic distribution, bilateral hilar hypermetabolic lymphadenopathy (MIP)

Breast cancer with positive right internal mammary lymph nodes

Diffuse lymphomatous pattern

1.2   Flash Facts: FDG PET/CT Findings Which Upstage Cancers

FDG PET/CT is an essential modality for the accurate staging of some cancers in which progression is suspected. FDG PET/CT utility is based on NCCN recommendation. A few key facts are important to remember when reading FDG PET/CT. The presence of these findings may affect patients' treatment and survival rate.

Lung (NSLC)
- *Mediastinal lymph nodes* (LN), ipsilateral or contralateral → *N2* → stage IIIA → *inoperable.*
- *Contralateral* lung, pleural/pericardial *effusion*, distant organ (look at the adrenals) *M1* → *stage IV.*

Breast
- Positive *internal mammary* lymph node → N2 → *stage IIIA* → *neoadjuvant chemotherapy.*

Pancreas
- Tumor involving the *celiac axis* or *superior mesenteric artery* → *T4* → stage III → *inoperable.*

Prostate (FDG PET/CT usually not recommended):
- *Positive LNs* → stage IV.

Endometrial Carcinoma
- Presence of *lymph nodes* (N1, N2), malignant *ascites*, peritoneal *implants* (M1) → *surgical debulking* +/- neoadjuvant chemotherapy.

Head and Neck Cancer
- *Direct invasion to the thyroid cartilage (laryngeal CA)*, floor of mouth, larynx, extrinsic muscle of tongue, medial pterygoid, hard palate (*oropharyngeal* cancer) → T4 → stage IV → *inoperable.*
- *Cervical LN >6 cm* → N3 → T4 → stage IV → *inoperable.*

Lymphoma
- Spread on *both sides of the diaphragm* or *splenic* involvement → *stage III*. Extra lymphatic involvement (except spleen) → stage 4 (stages III and IV → same treatment approach). Based on Ann Arbor staging.
- *Low-grade lymphomas (mild increased FDG uptake)*: Small lymphocyte B cell, marginal zone B cell, MALT, peripheral T cell lymphoma.
- *High-grade lymphomas (intense increased FDG uptake)*: Hodgkin's, diffuse large B cell, mantle lymphoma, follicular lymphoma.

Melanoma
- T → define by pathology (thickness and +/- ulceration). N → number of +LN (N1, 1 LN; N2, 2–3 LNs; N3, >4 LNs).

1.3   Lesions Without High FDG Uptake

Sclerotic bone lesions which may not show significant FDG uptake
- Prostate carcinoma.
- Breast carcinoma: Mixed sclerotic and lytic lesions – FDG PET/CT is widely used due to mixed pattern.
- Transitional cell carcinoma (TCC).
- Carcinoid bone lesions.
- Lymphoma.

Low cellular cancers with low FDG PET/CT sensitivity
- Mucinous cancers.
- Lung adenocarcinoma in situ.

Low glucose utilization
- Hepatoma (HCC).
- Prostate cancer (low grade).
- Low-grade neuroendocrine tumors.
- Low-grade lymphoma.

Suggested Reading
- Musculoskeletal; Bone Tumors; Henk Jan van de Woude and Robin Smithuis, Radiology department of the Onze Lieve Vrouwe Gasthuis, Amsterdam and the Rijnland hospital, Leiderdorp, Netherlands. http://www.radiologyassistant.nl/en

2 NaF

2.1 PET/CT Bone Imaging with F-18 NaF

Clinical Use Bone scan agent was FDA approved in 1972 and withdrawn in 1975 due to ready availability and low cost of Tc-99m PYP and, in 1978, Tc-MDP. In addition, PET scanners were in very few hospitals at that time. F-18 NaF requires institutional investigational new drug application (IND). Not reimbursable.

Other clinical use – non-FDA-approved (under research) identification of <u>active</u> coronary atherosclerosis.

F-18 Cyclotron produced. t_{phys} 109.8 min. *Decays* positron emission to O-18. 511 KeV photons are emitted (annihilation radiation).

Mechanism IV injection of F-18 NaF → chemisorption onto hydroxyapatite (rapid process) → exchange diffusion – the OH⁻ group on the hydroxyapatite exchanges with F-18 → forms fluorapatite (slower process – days to weeks).

Higher uptake will be within exposed bone surface (where mineralization accrues) such as in tumors, inflammation, post-trauma, and active process atherosclerosis.

Advantage: PET agent (higher spatial resolution), measures increase in regional blood flow (high first pass) and attached to exposed bone surface (uptake in both lytic and sclerotic lesions).

Image Protocol (Bone Oncology)

Prep.: (1) Hydration and (2) void prior to and after injection (decreases radiation dose to the bladder).

Image whole body: CT – for attenuation correction *PET* 45–60 min postinjection 2–5 min per bed positing.

Dose: 5–10 mCi.

Critical Organ Bone.

Distribution First pass of 100 % from the blood pool to bone capillaries which freely diffuses across the membranes. 1 h postinjection less than 10 % remains in the blood pool.

Clearance Rapidly cleared by the kidneys.

Suggested Reading

- Czernin J et al (2010). Molecular mechanisms of bone 18F-NaF deposition. J Nucl Med 51(12):1826–1829
- Derlin T et al (2010). Feasibility of 18F-sodium fluoride PET/CT for imaging of atherosclerotic plaque. J Nucl Med 51:862–865

Distribution and Clearance

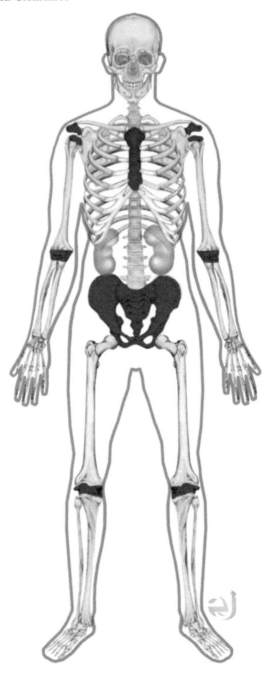

Distribution First pass of 100 % from the blood pool to bone capillaries, which freely diffuses across the membranes. 1 h postinjection, less than 10 % remains in the blood pool.
Clearance Rapidly cleared by the kidneys.

3   Rb-82

3.1   PET/CT Cardiac Imaging with Rb-82 Chloride

Indications Perfusion agent for cardiac PET stress scans.
1. Detection of coronary artery disease and myocardial perfusion abnormalities before and after interventional therapy.
2. Surgical risk evaluation.
3. Detection of hibernating myocardium in conjunction with F-18 fluorodeoxyglucose (FDG).

Rb-82 Generator-produced strontium-82/Rb-82 generator system.

t_{phys} 76 s. *Emits* annihilation photons 511 keV, prompts gamma (776 keV, 15 % abundance and 1395 keV, 0.5 % abundance). *Decays* 95 % by positron emission and 5 % by electron capture.

Mechanism Potassium analog – transports across the myocardial membrane via NA^+-K^+ ATPase.

First-Pass Extraction Rb-82: 61 % (tetrofosmin, 50 %; sestamibi, 60 %; Tl-201, 85–91 %).

Critical Organ Kidneys.

Imaging PET/CT of the chest.

Dose 40–60 mCi.

Imaging Protocol (1) CT scan for attenuation correction purposes. (2) Rb-82 IV over 30–60 s. (3) Image 2 min postinjection for 5 min. (4) 10 min postinjection stress images can be performed. (5) Viability study can be performed with FDG.

Distribution According to the cardiac output. 5 % coronary arteries and 20 % kidneys. Does not cross the BBB.

Clearance Myocardium, kidneys, thyroid, liver, and stomach.

Distribution and Clearance

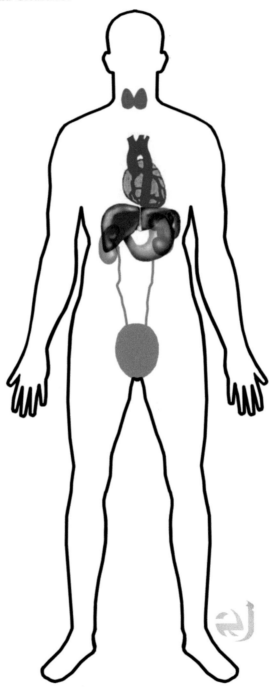

Distribution According to the cardiac output. 5 % coronary arteries and 20 % kidneys.
Clearance Myocardium, kidneys, thyroid, liver, and stomach.

Part 5: Clinical Nuclear Medicine – Multi-use Radiopharmaceuticals-Based Flash Facts

Contents

© Springer International Publishing Switzerland 2017
B. Savir-Baruch, B.J. Barron, *RadTool Nuclear Medicine Flash Facts*,
DOI 10.1007/978-3-319-24636-9_5

1   Tc-99m Tetrofosmin (Myoview)/Tc-99m Sestamibi (Cardiolite)

Indication Parathyroid adenoma, cardiac stress scan, breast cancer

Tc-99m Generator produced. Mo-99 _Generator_ → Tc-99m pertechnetate (TcO_4^{1-}) _undergoing isomeric transition_ → Tc-99 (half-life of 211,000 years) β-_decay_ → ruthenium-99. TcO_4^{1-} _Oxidation state of +7_ not suitable for medical applications. TcO_4^{1-} (+7) tetrofosmin/sestamibi _with Stannous ion_ → Tc-99m (+4 Tetrofosmin/+3 Sestamibi) → lipophilic, cationic Tc-99m complex. t_{phys} 6 h. _Emits_ gamma 140 KeV (89 %), 18.37 keV (4.0 %), 18.25 keV (2.1 %).

Mechanism Tetrofosmin/Sestamibi.

Lipophilic structure: Passive diffuse to the cell → uptake by mitochondria due to membrane electric potential → retention due to electrostatic interactions → trapped within the mitochondria.

Oxyphil cells: Secreting cell → higher mitochondria concentration → higher tracer retention.

Wash out by Pgp (P glycoprotein). Tumor cell [Pgp] expression is related to tumor multidrug resistance (breast CA).

Myocardium Uptake is proportional to blood flow. _First-pass extraction_ tetrofosmin 50 %, _sestamibi_ 60 %, _total myocardial uptake_ up to 2 % of the injected dose, _cardiac wash-out_ tetrofosmin>>sestamibi.

Parathyroid Parathyroid adenoma expression of oxyphil secretion cells is higher than normal thyroid gland. Parathyroid adenoma will show tracer retention on delay images.

Breast Cancer Mitochondrial expression is higher in malignant and inflammatory cells compare with benign cells. Only Tc-99m sestamibi is FDA approved for breast imaging. Known as Miraluma.

Distribution _Early 30 min_ Thyroid salivary gland, heart >>> liver, kidney.

Late >60 min Biliary tract, GI, kidney, bladder > liver, heart >> thyroid, salivary gland.

Clearance Bile to GI and kidney.

Distribution and Clearance

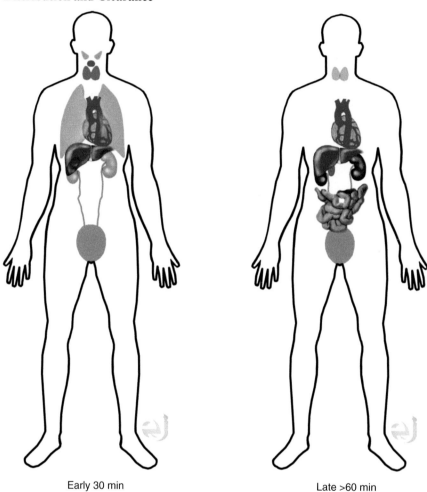

Early 30 min   Late >60 min

Distribution *Early 30 min* Thyroid salivary gland, heart > heart >>>liver, kidney.
      Late >60 min Biliary tract, GI, kidney, bladder >liver, heart >> thyroid, salivary gland.
Clearance Bile to GI and kidney.

2   Tl-201 Chloride

Indication   Cardiac stress test (perfusion agent for rest study in a dual isotope cardiac stress scan Tl-201/Tc-99 sestamibi) and viability (redistribution). Brain tumor or thyroid Ca localization (rarely used).

Tl-201   Cyclotron produced t_{phys} 73.1 h. For Tl chloride, t_{biol} 9.8 days, t_{eff} 2.4 days. *Decays* by Electron capture to Mercury (Hg-201), which *emits* X ray 69–80 KeV (94 %), gamma 135 keV (2.0 %), 167 keV (10 %).

First-Pass Extraction Rate   85–91 % (tetrofosmin 50 %, sestamibi 60 %) *Total myocardial uptake* is 3 % of the injected dose. Peak at 10 min.

Mechanism   Potassium analog; transports across the myocardial membrane via NA$^+$-K$^+$ ATPase. Perfusion agent. Does not cross blood-brain barrier (BBB). Can be used for tumor localization scan – BBB breakdown → increase uptake of tracer by tumor cells.

Redistribution   Dynamic exchange of Tl-201 between circulation and intracellular.

Viability Study   *Delayed imaging:* Tracer redistribution in a fixed defect → presence of hibernating tissue → patient will benefit from revascularization.

Brain Tumors   Usually used to differentiate brain lesions from lymphoma and infection in HIV/AIDS patients. Positive uptake → lymphoma.

Imaging   20 % window 80 KeV peak.

Protocol Cardiac   Rest component of the Tc-99m dual study. (1) Fasting for 4 h. (2) Inject 3–3.5 mCi Tl-201 IV (3) after 10 min SPECT images 64 frames 20 % window for 80 KeV peak. (4) Stress images with Tc-99 MIBI/Myoview. (5) If fixed defect → delayed SPECT images with 20 % window 80 KeV peak for redistribution.

Protocol Brain   planar images followed by SPECT.

Dose   *Cardiac scan* 3–3.5 mCi. *Brain* 5.0 mCi.

Critical Organ   Testes in males, kidneys in females.

Distribution   According to the cardiac output. 5 % coronary arteries, 20 % kidneys. Does not cross BBB.

Clearance   Myocardium, kidneys, thyroid, liver, and stomach.

Distribution and Clearance

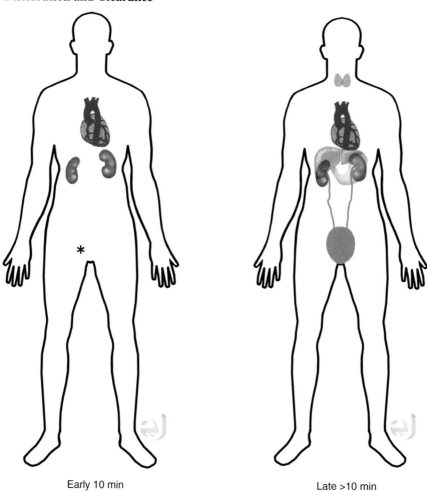

Early 10 min   Late >10 min

Distribution According to the cardiac output. 5% Coronary arteries, 20% Kidneys. Does
        not cross BBB.
Clearance Myocardium, kidneys, thyroid, liver, and stomach.
* Testicular uptake.

3   Tc-99m Sulfur Colloid (SC)

Indications
1. Lymphoscintigraphy – Localization of sentinel lymph node (breast cancer, melanoma), and lymphedema.
2. Liver/spleen scan – Evaluation of liver function.
3. Diagnosis of focal nodular hyperplasia (FNH).
4. Bone marrow (BM) scan – Evaluation of BM reticuloendothelial system (RES).
5. Gastroesophageal reflux (GER) studies.
6. Gastric emptying study.
7. Pulmonary aspiration studies.
8. Peritoneovenous (LeVeen) shunt patency.
9. Cystography.
10. Dacryoscintigraphy.

Tc-99m Generator produced in the form of Tc 99m pertechnetate (TcO_4^{1-}) (+7 valence) from Mo-99. t_{phys} 6 h. *Emits* gamma 140 KeV (89 %), 18.37 KeV (4.0 %), 18.25 KeV (2.1 %).

Sulfur Colloid particles size of 0.1–2.0 μm before filtration; 0.1–0.2 μm after filtration for lymphoscintigraphy.

Tc-99m SC Preparation kit *does not include stannous ion* to bind TcO_4^{1-} with SC. The *only* tracer that does not require stannous.

Mechanism of Action
- *IV admin*: SC particles will be taken via phagocytosis to the RES and will be trapped.
- *Subcutaneous/intradermal*: SC particles will be extracted by subcutaneous lymphatic system (phagocytosis) to regional LNs.
- *Oral:* GI distribution.

Protocol See separate dedicated scan cards.

Dose
- *Lymphoscintigraphy* 0.1 to 1 mCi.
- *Liver/spleen* 1 to 8 mCi; typical dose ~ 5 mCi.
- *Bone marrow scan* 3 to 12 mCi.
- *Gastroesophageal scan* 0.15 to 0.30 mCi and pulmonary aspiration studies by oral route 0.30 to 0.50 mCi.
- *Peritoneovenous (LeVeen) shunt patency* intraperitoneal injection 1 to 3 mCi; percutaneous transtubal injection 0.3 to 1 mCi.
- *Via Foley* adult 1–2 mCi; child (5 years old) 0.5–1.0 mCi.

Target Organ *IV*: liver. *subcutaneous*: injection site. *oral*: large intestine.

Distribution *IV admin*: 85 % liver Kupffer cells (phagocytes), spleen macrophages, (10 %) and bone marrow (5 %). *Subcutaneous/intradermal:* SC particles will be extract by the lymphatic system to regional LNs. *Oral*: GI distribution

Clearance *IV and SC:* via phagocytosis – Tc-99m sulfur colloid particles will be fixed intracellularly. *Oral*: Not absorbed, fecal excretion. *Via Foley:* bladder emptying.

Distribution Patterns

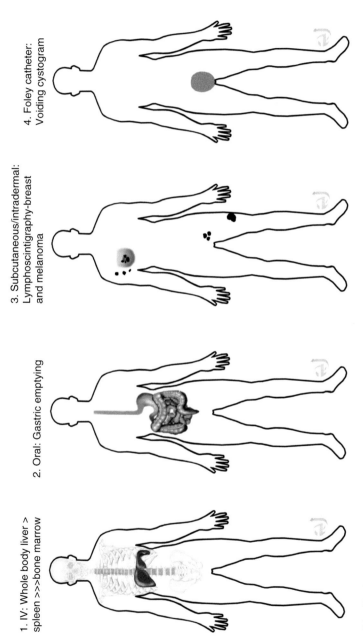

1. IV: Whole body liver > spleen >>>bone marrow

2. Oral: Gastric emptying

3. Subcutaneous/intradermal: Lymphoscintigraphy-breast and melanoma

4. Foley catheter: Voiding cystogram

Distribution: IV admin: 85% liver Kupffer cells (phagocytes), spleen macrophages, (10%) and bone marrow (5%). **Subcutaneous/intradermal:** SC particles will be extract by the lymphatic system to regional LNs. **Oral:** GI distribution **Via Foley** Urinating.

Clearance: IV and SC: Via phagocytosis- Tc-99m sulfur colloid particles will be fixed intracellularly. **Oral:** Not absorbed, Fecal excretion. **Via Foley** Bladder emptying.

4   Tc-99m Pertechnetate

Indications Evaluation of Meckel's diverticulum, evaluation of thyroid nodules, GI bleeding (not commonly used), perfusion tracer (brain death, veins and central lines patency, first pass for cardiac images), and dacryoscintigraphy.

Tc-99m Generator produced. Molybdenum-99 (Mo-99) *Generator* (half-life of 66 h) elutes Tc-99m (TcO$_4$^{1}). t_{phys} 6 h. *Emits* gamma 140 KeV (89 %).

Meckel's Diverticulum Ectopic gastric mucosa that might bleed.

Mechanism: Tc-99m Pertechnetate will be rapidly absorbed and secreted by mucous cells of the gastric mucosa. Rapid gastric uptake will be noted. In the presence of gastric mucosa within a Meckel's diverticulum, an area of Tc-99m TcO$_4$$^{1-}$ uptake will be seen. H2 blocker prior to the exam → minimized abnormal secretion of tracer by the gastric mucosa → decreased accumulation of traced gastric mucous → decreased false-positive studies.

Protocol: _Patient preparation_ – Fasting 4 h prior. Crushed cimetidine 20 mg/kg orally 30 min prior to the exam. _Dose_: Children – 30–100 μCi/kg (minimum of 200 μCi). Adults 10 mCi. _Imaging_: 1 min flow (60, 1 s/frame). Static images every 5–10 min for 1 h or dynamic images, an image every 60 s x 60 min.

Interpretation: Positive study will demonstrate an ectopic focus of increased uptake in the abdomen.

Thyroid Scan

Mechanism: Tc-99m TcO$_4$$^{1-}$ will pass via the I/Na symporter channel the thyroid follicles without organification. Role in thyroid scanning: Evaluation of thyroid agenesis/lingual thyroid in neonates with hypothyroidism. If thyroid uptake is noted in the thyroid bed → evaluate for organification failure with I-123 scan. Thyroid nodules: decreased uptake (cold nodule) of Tc-99m TcO$_4$$^{1-}$ (15–20 % chance of malignancy) → Biopsy. If increased uptake is noted on TcO$_4$$^{1-}$ (hot nodule) → perform I-123 scan → If no uptake → discordant nodule (positive on Tc-99m and negative on I-123 scans) → Biopsy.

Protocol: Patient preparation – stop antithyroid medication. Dose: 5 mCi IV. Image: LEHR collimator anterior images. Pinhole images in ANT RAO and LAO projections.

Perfusion Images

Can be used as first-pass perfusion tracer similar to arterial phase on CT scans (CTA), to examine brain perfusion for the evaluation of brain death (see brain death chapter), or to evaluate atrial, venous, and line patency.

Protocol: image 1 s/frame for 1 min of the desired region. Now with the advantage of CT imaging, this study is rarely performed.

Pitfall Diffuse homogenous increased gastric uptake in Ultratag RBC GI bleed scan likely to demonstrate free Tc-99m due to poor labeling.

Target organ: Kidney.

Distribution Thyroid, salivary gland, stomach, and kidney.

Clearance Kidneys → bladder.

Distribution and Clearance

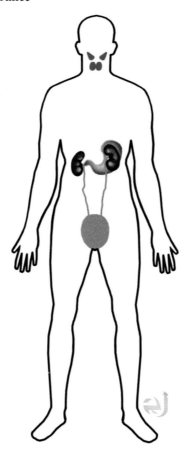

Distribution Thyroid, salivary gland, stomach, kidney
Clearance Kidneys → bladder

Distribution and Clearance

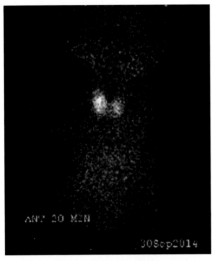

Thyroid uptake in infant

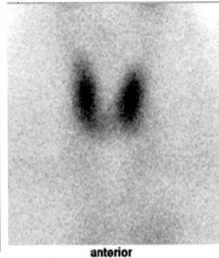

anterior
Thyroid uptake in Adult

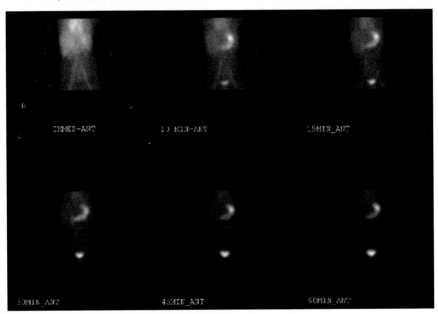

Normal distribution of Tc-99m TcO_4^{1-}

Abnormal Distribution Patterns

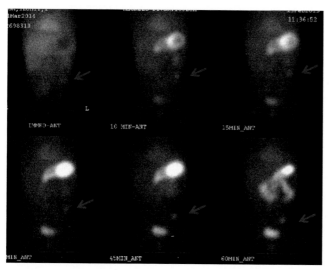

Positive scan with uptake in an ectopic gastric mucosa within the left lower abdomen in a young child, stable in location throughout the study (if motion is noted – will support GI contamination from gastric tracer secretion or active GI bleeding.

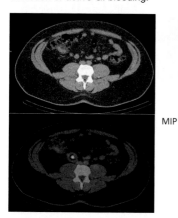

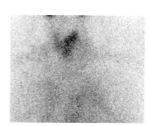

MIP

Hyperthyroidism with enlarge left thyroid lobe.

Localization of positive Meckel's scan for ectopic gastric mucosa, using SPECT/CT in adult.

5   Ceretec© (Tc-99m HMPAO) Tc-99m Hexamethylpropyleneamine Oxime

Indications
Cerebral flow and perfusion (dementia, epilepsy, and brain death).
Preparation of tagged WBC (infection).
Tc-99m Generator produced in the form of Tc-99m pertechnetate (TcO_4^{1-}) from Mo-99. t_{phys} 6 h. *Emits* gamma 140 KeV (89 %).
Tc-99m HMPAO Lipophilic structure, crosses BBB, first-pass extraction of roughly 80 %.

Mechanism
Cerebral flow: Blood pool → crosses BBB (lipophilic) → intracellular (cortical cell, via glutathione) → convert to hydrophilic complex → trapped → taken by the mitochondria and the nucleus. For brain death scan, blue dye is used to stabilize the molecule. It prevents the conversion of the Tc-99m HMPAO to a stereoisomerism form that rapidly washes out from the brain tissue.
WBC tagged: Ceretec – WBC complex → will follow the WBC distribution.

Dose
Cerebral flow: 20 mCi.
Tagged WBC: 20 mCi.

Protocol
Brain perfusion/flow: Inject 20 mCi of Ceretec → 15 min–2 h post injection SPECT as close as possible to the head.
Tagged WBC: Patient prep – wound dressing change → 50 ml autologous blood → WBC separation → prepare 20 mCi dose of Tc-99m WBC → reinjection → image at 30 min (up to 2 h) for intra-abdominal /inflammatory bowel disease or at 4 h for other infections followed by 24 h delayed images as needed.

Critical Organ *Cerebral flow*: lacrimal glands. *Tagged WBC:* spleen.

Distribution *Brain perfusion*: Trapped in brain (intracellular, trapped); muscle and soft tissue (none trapped).
Tagged WBC: Spleen > liver >> bowel, bone marrow, kidney, gallbladder, some lung.

Clearance *Brain perfusion*: decays in the brain (trapped). Kidneys and hepatobiliary (non-trapped). *Tagged WBC:* Renal > hepatobiliary.

Distribution and Clearance

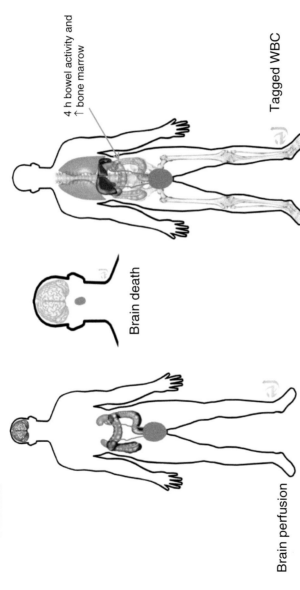

4 h bowel activity and ↑ bone marrow

Brain death

Brain perfusion

Tagged WBC

Distribution *Brain perfusion* Trapped in brain (intracellular, trapped), muscle and soft tissue (none trapped). **Tagged WBC** Spleen > liver >> bowel, bone marrow, kidney, gallbladder, some lung.

Clearance *Brain perfusion* decays in the brain (trapped). Kidneys and hepatobiliary (non-trapped). **Tagged WBC:** Renal > hepatobiliary.

Distribution and Clearance

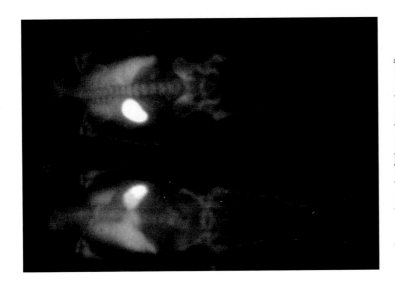

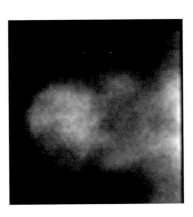

Distribution *Brain perfusion* Trapped in brain (intracellular, trapped), muscle and soft tissue (none trapped).

Tagged WBC Spleen > liver >> bowel, bone marrow, kidney, gallbladder, some lung.

Clearance *Brain perfusion* decays in the brain (trapped). Kidneys and hepatobiliary (non-trapped). **Tagged WBC:** Renal > hepatobiliary.

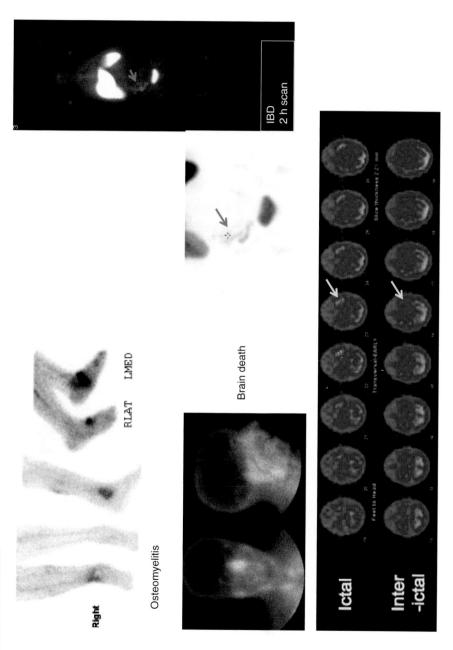

Part 6: Nuclear Medicine – Radionuclide Therapies

Contents

1   Thyroid Ablation

1.1   Thyroid Ablation with I-131 Na. Low-Dose Treatment <33 mCi

Indications Clinical and subclinical hyperthyroidism (low TSH).

I-131 Fission product. t_{phys} 8.1 days *Emits* gamma photons 364.4 KeV and β-energy. *Thyroid radiation dose* approximately 1 rad/μCi.

I- 123 Cyclotron-produced t_{phys} 13.3 h *Emits* gamma photons 159 KeV.

Mechanism Rapid GI absorption of iodine to the extracellular fluid → active uptake in the thyroid follicles by Na/I symport (trapping) → protein bound iodine (organification). All drugs which affect the thyroid hormone synthesis pathway will affect iodine uptake (highly regulated by TSH). Additional uptake (nonprotein-bounded uptake mechanism) by salivary gland, stomach cells (no trapping), and hepatocytes (thyroglobulin metabolism).

Thyroid Uptake Evaluation

Preparation Stop Tapazole (methimazole) and PTU for 3 days; no iodinated contrast study in the last 6 weeks. Stop amiodarone 3–6 m prior to treatment.

Perform pregnancy test (when applicable) using urine or serum test, ideally within 24 h prior treatment.

Diagnostic Dose with I-123 NaI

Day 1 0.2–0.4 mCi of I-123 NaI oral uptake.

Day 2 Thyroid scan and uptake.

Ablation Dose with I-131 NaI (*Written directive is required, signed by an authorized user*).

Method 1: **Formula based: Dose will be calculated based on % thyroid gland uptake and thyroid mass.**

$$Dose\,(mCi) = \frac{\text{Thyroid Mass(g)} \times 0.08 - 0.22(mCi/g)}{\text{Thyroid Uptake(\%)}} \times 100 \,(\%)$$

Range is typically 6–30 mCi.

Method 2: Empiric dose for Graves' disease, toxic multinodular goiter, and solitary toxic nodules. 15 (toxic nodule) −30 mCi (multinodular goiter).

Day of treatment: Check for pregnancy test results when applicable. Sign an agreement for therapy consent. Call to order (dose, name of the patient, and date of birth). Give the capsule with one glass of water. Hold food and liquids for 2 h.

Follow up with endocrinology for TSH level.

1.2 Thyroid Ablation with I-131 NaI. High-Dose Treatment >33 mCi

Preparation

Target TSH level: >30 μU/mL (achieved by Thyrogen IM injections or withdrawal of Synthroid). No iodinated contrast study in the last 6–8 weeks.

Low iodine diet: 10–14 days before administration of therapy. Stop low iodine diet 2 h up to 72 h after treatment (no definitive consensus).

Pregnancy test: (when applicable) using urine or serum test, ideally within 24 h prior treatment.

Ablation Protocols

<u>Surveillance protocol</u> indicated when patient has low thyroglobulin level after prior ablation.

<u>Day 1</u> Thyrogen 0.9 mg IM.

<u>Day 2</u> Thyrogen 0.9 mg IM.

<u>Day 2 or 3</u> 4 mCi of I-131 NaI or 2 mCi of I-123 NaI.

<u>Day 4 or 5</u> Whole body scan at 48 h after the oral uptake of I-131 NaI or at 24 h after the oral uptake of I-123 NaI.

If treatment is indicated, repeat with treatment protocol.

<u>Treatment protocol</u> indicated when patient has high thyroglobulin level after prior ablation or 2–3 months after thyroidectomy.

Thyrogen (recombinant TSH) injection protocol

<u>Day 1</u> Thyrogen IM.

<u>Day 2</u> Thyrogen IM + *NaI-123* oral uptake.

<u>Day 3</u> Whole body scan followed by treatment with I-131 NaI as needed (ideally I-131 NaI treatment will be given when TSH peaks at 36 h post 2nd Thyrogen injection).

Withdrawal protocol

Patient preparation: Discontinue thyroid hormone – T_4 (thyroxine) for 3–4 weeks, T_3 (triiodothyronine) 10–14 days, until *TSH > 30 μU/mL.*

<u>Day 1</u> I-123 NaI 2 mCi (may also use I-131 NaI 2–4 mCi).

<u>Day 2 or day 3</u> Whole body scan at 48 h after the oral uptake of I-131 NaI or at 24 h after the oral uptake of I-123 NaI.

<u>Treatment:</u> As long as patient is off thyroid hormones, treatment can be given on any day. Resume thyroid replacement hormones 72 h posttreatment.

TSH Suppression Posttreatment

High-risk and intermediate-risk thyroid cancer patients: TSH < 0.1 mU/L.

Low risk patients: TSH 0.1–0.5 mU/L.

Dose

Diagnostic Dose with I-123 NaI

    0.2–0.4 mCi of I-123 NaI oral uptake.

Ablation dose with I-131 NaI

Will be based on I-123 distribution and pathology report.

    Local disease (thyroid bed): 30–100 mCi I-131 NaI (the higher the uptake in the thyroid surgical bed, the lower the ablation dose).

    Positive LNs: 150–200 mCi I-131 NaI.

    Metastasis: $\geq$200 mCi I-131 NaI.

Lung metastasis will be based on dosimetry to prevent long-term pulmonary fibrosis; limit of 80 mCi/2.96 GBq activity retention in the lung (George Sgouros et al., J Nucl Med. 2006;47(12):1977–1984).

Safety Negative pregnancy test (when applicable).

Critical Organ Thyroid.

Distribution Iodine containing tissue (thyroid tissue, salivary gland, sebaceous glands, and stomach), GI lumen (oral admin), 7 days post therapy scan may demonstrate liver uptake due to circulating thyroglobulin. Thyroglobulin will be metabolized by the hepatocytes.

Clearance By kidneys, metabolized in the liver.

Suggested Reading

- Society of nuclear medicine procedure guideline for therapy of thyroid disease with iodine-131 (sodium iodide) 3.0
- Bryan R. Haugen et al; 2015 American Thyroid Association Management Guidelines for Adult Patients with Thyroid Nodules and Differentiated Thyroid Cancer. The American Thyroid Association Guidelines Task Force on Thyroid Nodules and Differentiated Thyroid Cancer.

Distribution and Clearance

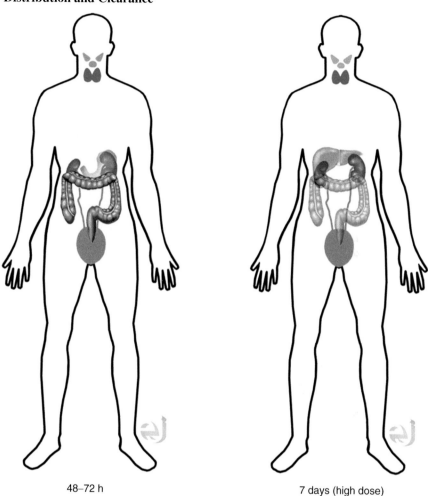

48–72 h   7 days (high dose)

Distribution Iodine containing tissue (thyroid tissue, salivary gland, and stomach)+GI lumen (oral admin), 7 days post scan – liver uptake due to thyroid hormone metabolism.
Clearance By kidneys, metabolized in the liver.

Distribution and Clearance

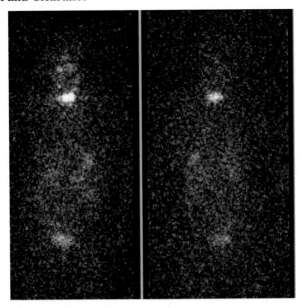

48–72 h I-131 4 mCi

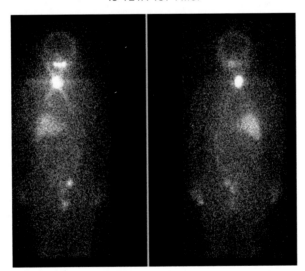

7 days I-131 150 mCi

Distribution Iodine containing tissue (thyroid tissue, salivary gland, and stomach)+GI lumen (oral admin), 7 days post scan – liver uptake due to thyroid hormone metabolism.

Clearance By kidneys, metabolized in the liver.

Abnormal Distribution Patterns

7 days post ablation-Iodine
concentration in liver cyst, benign

Pre ablation-LN, lung and sacral metastasis

2   Liver Tumor Ablation

2.1   Radioembolization with Yttrium-90 Microspheres

Indication Ablation of hepatocellular carcinoma and metastatic disease to the liver
Y-90 Pure β-emitter with bremsstrahlung radiation produced and detectable externally.
Y-90 production bombardment of Y-89 from nuclear reactor. Decays into stable zirconium. t_{phys} 64.1 h. *Emits: β-* with maximum energy of 2.284 MeV. *Average penetration*:
~ 5 mm in soft tissue (100–200 cells) *Images* : Y-90 low E Bremsstrahlung X-rays.
Microspheres
- *TheraSpheres* ® – Glass, FDA approved for unresectable HCC. Size: 20–30 μm,
  I mg contains 22,000–73,000 microspheres. Dose: 3 GBq (81 mCi) – 1.2 M
  microspheres, 5 GBq (135 mCi)–2 M, 7 GBq (189 mCi)–2.8 M, 10 GBq
  (270 mCi)–4 M, 15 GBq (405 mCi)–6 M, and 20 GBq (540 mCi)–8 M. Also can
  order a specific required dose. Activity per microsphere is approximately 2500 Bq.
- *SIR-Spheres* ® – Resin-based microspheres, 20–40 μm in diameter. FDA
  approved for colorectal liver metastasis. Dose: Vial of 3 GBq Y-90 in 5 mL of
  sterile water with 40–80 M microspheres. Activity per microsphere is
  approximately 50 Bq → higher number of particles will be adminis-
  trated → increased risk of particle clots.

Mechanism Hepatic tumors are predominantly perfused by the branches of the
hepatic artery (>90 %), while the hepatocytes are predominantly perfused by the
portal vein (>70–80 %). Microspheres are larger than the capillaries. Hence, once
injected via the selected branch of the hepatic artery, microspheres will be trapped
within capillary bed of the tumor.

Dose Per treatment planning protocol. Tumor radiation up to 50–150 Gy. Activity
per microsphere: SIR-Spheres – 50 Bq TheraSpheres- 2500 Bq.

Protocol *Preparation* (1) History, physical, and liver MRI (2) labs (CBC, chemistry, INR, LFT, PT, PTT, AFP, CEA).
- *Lung study shunt with Tc-99m MAA particles. Goal*: To assess lung and systemic
  shunting and to predict the coverage of live tumor masses by Y-90. IR radiologist
  will commonly coil the gastroduodenal artery (GDA) to prevent spread of Y-90
  to stomach. Followed by direct injection of Tc-99m MAA via the common
  hepatic artery. MAA particles will be trapped and reflect the arterial distribution → planar images → lung shunt will be calculated. SPECT/CT → assess for
  extrahepatic distribution and tumor coverage by the MAA (will predict the distribution of Y-90). *Dose calculation:* Decrease dose with increase lung shunt
  (20 % shunt may be used as the upper limit for treatment). Upper dose limit to
  the lung is 30 Gy in a single treatment and 50 Gy life time.
- *Y-90 treatment:* administration of Y-90 particles guided by fluoroscopy is via the
  selected branch of hepatic artery (right, left or segmental artery) – followed by
  Bremsstrahlung images. *Optional*: Fuse available FDG PET/CT with bremsstrahlung SPECT and with MRI to compare actual tumor uptake to planned distribution.

Pitfall As Y-90 is given via anatomical distribution (not tumor receptor based);
treatment should be given to one lobe at a time to prevent liver failure.

Distribution and Clearance

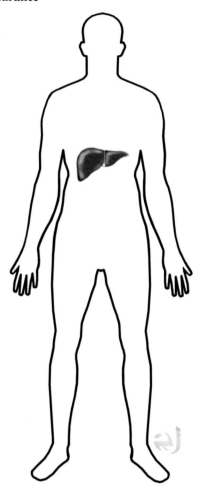

Tc-99m MAA or Y-90 microspheres injected via the selected branch of the hepatic artery will be trapped and will reflect the arterial distribution within the tumor capillary bed.

Yttrium-90 Radioembolization

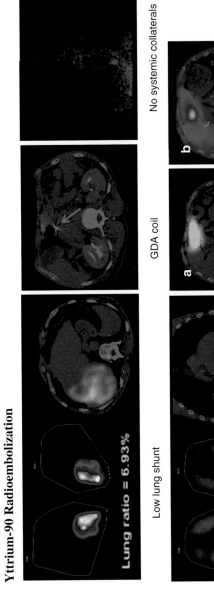

No systemic collaterals

GDA coil

Low lung shunt

Lung ratio = 6.93%

Lung shunt >20 %-patient is not a
candidate for treatment

Lung ratio = 48.69%

Fused MAA (a) and bremsstrahlung
SPECT/CT images (b)

3 Ablation of Bone Metastases

3.1 Palliation of Pain Caused by Bone Metastases: Beta-Minus Emitters

Indications Bone pain associated with diffuse metastases and are positive on bone scan.

Radiopharmaceuticals *Sm-153:* Samarium-153 EDTMP (ethylenediaminetetramethylene phosphonate), *Sr-89:* Strontium – 89 chloride, *P-32:* P-32 sodium phosphate.

Mechanism of Action Bone seeking agents act like phosphonates. Will be most effective during active bone remodeling with high amorphous calcium phosphate matrix, as in sclerotic lesions. P-32 distributes to bone due to its high inorganic phosphorus content. Sr-89 is a chemical analog of calcium.

Protocol Patient preparation: Hydration. Sm-153: radiation safety instruction (gamma-emitter). IV injection. Eligibility criteria: WBC >2400 and platelets >60,000. Schedule CBC follow-up at 6 weeks.

Myelosupression P-32 > Sr-89 > Sm-153. P-32 : 30–100 % of patients. Nadir is 4–5 weeks post-therapy. Recovery 6–7 weeks. Sr-89: 80 % of patients, Nadir is 5–6 weeks post therapy, recovery at 12 weeks. Sm-153: mild myelosuppression; Nadir is 4 weeks post therapy, recovery at 4–8 weeks.

Radionuclide	Target	Method of production	Decay product	Chemical form	Dose (mCi)	t_{phys} (days)	Max E (MeV)	Max range (mm)	Pain relief	Other
Sr-89	Sr-88	Thermal neutron reactor	Y-89	Chloride	4 mCi or 40–60 µCi/ kg	50.5	1.46 (β^-)	8	2 weeks up to 9 m. 10 % flare response	–
	Y-89	Fast reactor								
Sm-153	Varies	Nuclear reactor	Eu-153	EDTMP (Quadramet)	1.0 mCi/kg	1.95	0.81 (β^-)	3.4	7–21 days – up to 14 m. 10–20 % flare response	γ Photon 103 Kev (26 %)
P-32 (first agent)	N/A	Fast neutron reactor	S-32	Orthophosphate	7	14.3	1.71 (β^-)	8.5	14 days up to 5 m. 10 % flare response	Used to treat P Vera and serosal implants

3.2 Palliation of Pain Caused by Bone Metastases: Alpha Emitter Ra-223 Chloride (Xofigo)

Indications Bone pain associated with diffuse bone metastasis in patients with prostate cancer.

Radiopharmaceutical Radium-223 chloride. Xofigo is prepared from an Ac-227/Ra-223 Generator. t_{phys} 11.4 days

Mechanism of Action Ra-223 is a radioactive isotope of radium (group 2 in the periodic table, same as Ca and Sr). Ra-223 is a Ca analog which will bind to the hydroxyapatite bone matrix. Sclerotic lesions will increase bone turnover with increased bone matrix production → increased uptake of Ra-223. Only bone pain palliation agent to demonstrate increase in life expectancy. Average life extension is ~3 months.

Protocol *Dose:* 1.35 μCi/kg (50 Kbq/kg).

Administration: Slow IV injection over 1 min every 4 weeks for six treatments.
Patient eligibility requirements prior to first treatment: Absolute neutrophil count > 1.5 × 10^9/L, platelet count > 100 × 10^9/L, hemoglobin > 10 g/dl. *Patient eligibility requirements for subsequent treatments (#2 to #6):* Absolute neutrophil count > 1.0 × 10^9/L, platelet count > 50 × 10^9/L.

Target Organ Osteogenic cell (hydroxyapatite matrix).

Side Effects Nausea > diarrhea > vomiting > myelosuppression (pancytopenia, anemia, lymphocytopenia, thrombocytopenia, leukopenia, neutropenia).

Contraindication Metastasis to soft tissue

Advantage Xofigo studies revealed interval increase in overall median survival rate of 3 months.

Distribution *Xofigo* Bone >>>>> > Bowel.

Clearance Rapidly via the bowel. At 4 h post injection 61 % in the bone and 39 % in the bowel.

Distribution Patterns

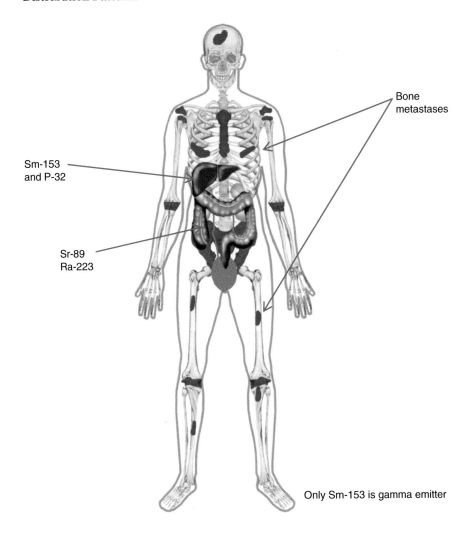

Bone
metastases

Sm-153
and P-32

Sr-89
Ra-223

Only Sm-153 is gamma emitter

Distribution Skeleton. Normal bone <<<<< Metastasis. *Sm-153* Skeleton >>> Liver (2–13 %), *P-32* Skeleton (85 %) >>> Liver. *Ra-223 and Sr-89* Bone >>>>>> Bowel

Clearance Kidneys: all beta emitters. Bowel: Xofigo. *Sr-89* Kidneys (approx. 66–80 %, 2 days peak), GI (34–20 %) *Sm-153* Kidneys (completed by 6 h.) *P-32* Kidneys (>85 % reabsorbed. Secreted over weeks). Xofigo rapidly via the bowel (At 4 h. 61 % in the bone and 39 % in the bowel).

4 Lymphoma Ablation

4.1 Bexxar I-131 Tositumomab

Production was terminated by the company.

Indication CD20 receptor positive, follicular, non-Hodgkin's lymphoma (NHL) with and without transformation, refractory to Rituximab and has relapsed following chemotherapy.

Bexxar treatment response 63 %; effects on survival is not known.

I-131 t_{phys} 8 days, *Decays* β- (606 KeV); *gamma ray energy:* 364 KeV *Production:* fission reactor.

Tositumomab Murine IgG2a monoclonal antibody against CD20. CD20 primarily expressed on late pro B cells and will be expressed until last stage of maturation (will not be expressed on plasma cell).

Mechanism I-131-Tositumomab targets CD20 expressed cells in NHL → radioablation of attached WBC.

Protocol Murine monoclonal antibodies (any subtype) can induce HAMA (human anti-mouse antibody); elevation leads to immune reaction. Therefore, HAMA level should be checked prior to injection.

Day before: Start thyroid block with SSKI (saturated potassium iodide) or Lugol's solution and continue for 2 weeks after injection: Block iodide uptake by the thyroid due to dissociation from the Bexxar.

Day 1: (1) Pretreat with Tylenol (pain), Benadryl (allergy) and tositumomab 450 mg over 1 h (block excess CD20 sites). (2) I-131 Bexxar 5 mCi over 20 min. (3) 1st dosimetry scan after 1 h of infusion and prior to urination.

Day 2, 3 or 4: 2nd dosimetry *scan* post void – view biodistribution.

Day 6 or 7: 3rd dosimetry *scan* post void – view biodistribution and calculate dose.

Day 7–14 (therapy day): (1) pre-treat with Tositumomab 450 mg over 1 h. (2) Therapy dose Bexxar over 20 min (90–150 mCi) injected through IV catheter with a 0.2 mm filter.

Discharge home: Radiation < 500 mrem exposure to others.

Dose

Platelet > 150 k 75 cGy in mCi.

100 k ≤ platelet ≤ 150 k 65 cGy in mCi.

Formula: Iodine-131 Activity (mCi) = [activity hr (mCi h)/residence time (h)] × [desired total body dose (cGy)/75 cGy]

Activity h: Patient's maximum effective mass derived from the patient's sex and height.

Residence Time (H.): Geometric mean of count taken from the dosimetry scans (three scans).

Toxicity Transfusion and colony stimulating (15 %), hypothyroidism, rare: myelo-dysplastic or leukemia and HAMA reaction.

Critical Organ Thyroid.

Distribution

1st scan (1 h pre-void): Most of the activity is in the blood pool >>>>> liver and spleen.

2nd and 3rd scan (>72 h post-void): ↓↓↓blood pool (BP) < ↓↓liver and spleen < thyroid, kidney, and urinary bladder and minimal uptake in the lungs.

Altered Biodistribution

1st scan: No blood pool.

1st, 2nd, and 3rd scan: Suggestive of GU obstruction, liver, and spleen↑↑↑>>>> BP, or lung >>> BP.

3rd scan: Total body residence times of less than 50 h or more than 150 h.

Clearance Kidney >>> bowel.

Distribution and Clearance

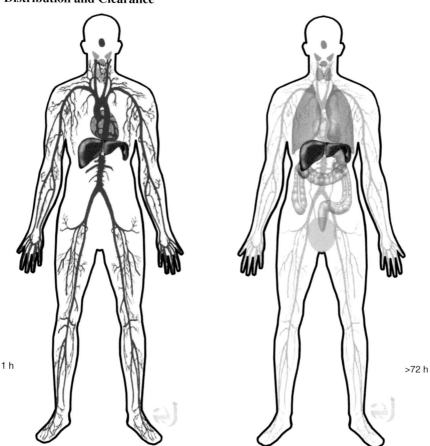

1 h   >72 h

Distribution

1st Scan (1 h pre-void): Most of the activity will be in the blood pool >>>>> liver and spleen.

2nd and 3rd scan (>72 h post-void): ↓↓↓blood pool (BP)<↓↓liver and spleen<thyroid, kidney, and urinary bladder and minimal uptake in the lungs.

Clearance *Kidney >>> Bowel*

4.2   Y-90 Zevalin Y-90 Ibritumomab Tiuxetan

Indication Treatment of follicular low-grade non-Hodgkin's lymphoma (refractory to Rituximab, relapsed or transformed)

Y-90 Pure β- emitter with bremsstrahlung radiation produced and detectable externally. *Y-90 production* bombardment of Y-89 in a nuclear reactor; decays into stable zirconium. t_{phys} 64.1 h

Emits β-maximum energy 2.284 MeV.

Penetration Average of 5 mm in soft tissue (100–200 cells)

Images Y-90 low E bremsstrahlung X-ray detection

Zevalin Y-90 labeled Murine anti-CD20 monoclonal antibody ibritumomab (by chelating agent Tiuxetan)

Mechanism of Action Targets CD 20 antigen in the surface of normal and tumor B cells.

Protocol *Day 1* Rituximab 250 mg/m²

  Days 7–9 Rituximab 250 mg/m² follow by IV Y-90 Zevalin at ≥ 4 h

Dose Based on patient weight and platelet count:

  0.4 mCi/kg (~15 MBq/kg) for patients with platelets >150 K

  0.3 mCi/kg (~11 MBq/kg) for patients with platelets between 100 and 150 K

  Maximal dose of 32 mCi due to possible bone marrow irradiation secondary to dissociation of Y-90 from the Zevalin molecule

Contraindication Platelets below 100,000; >25 % bone marrow involvement; known reaction to Murine Ab. Check human anti-mouse IgG antibody (HAMA) levels.

Side Effects 7–9 weeks : (1) cytopenia – neutrophil, Plt, Hgb. Last from 7 to 35 days. (2) Bleeding – thrombocytopenia. (3) Aggressive lymphoma/AML

Distribution Blood pool up to 96 h. Liver, spleen >>> bone marrow (if involved) and blood pool

Clearance Kidney >>> Bowel

Distribution and Clearance

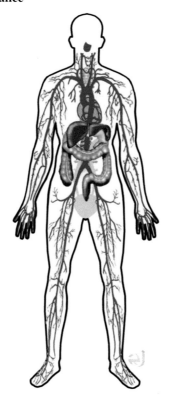

Distribution Blood pool up to 96 h. Liver, spleen >>> bone marrow (if involved) and blood pool
Clearance Kidney >>> Bowel

Ablation Effect

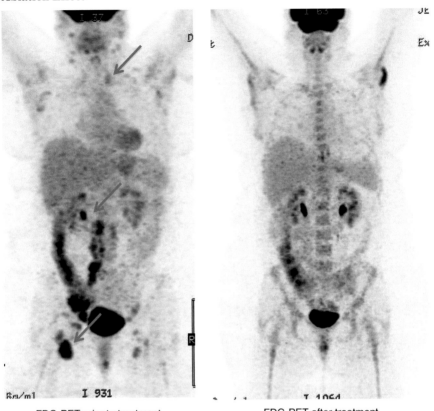

FDG-PET prior to treatment   FDG-PET after treatment

5 Neuroendocrine Tumor Ablation

5.1 I-131 MIBG

Clinical Use Treatment of widespread tumors that arise in neuroectodermal tissues (pheochromocytomas, neuroblastomas, carcinoid tumors, medullary thyroid tumors, paragangliomas, and chemodectomas).
I-131 t_{phys} 8.1 days, *Decays* β-(606 KeV), *gamma ray energy*: 364 keV *Production*: fission reaction
MIBG MetaIodoBenzylGuanidine (Iobenguane) norepinephrine analog.
I-123 MIBG: Use for localization and pre- and post I-131 high-dose treatment evaluation.
I-131 MIBG: Mainly use for neuroendocrine tumor ablation (high dose) and can be used for localization (low dose).
Mechanism: Norepinephrine analogue. Taken up as cytoplasmic synaptic vesicles by the presynaptic adrenergic axons via type I energy-dependent, active amine transport mechanism.
Protocol
Patient preparation
Medication to be stopped prior to exam
　Tricyclic antidepressants and related drugs – avoid for 6 weeks.
　Antihypertensives (Ca channel blocker, labetolol, reserpine) – avoid 2 weeks.
　Sympathetic amines (pseudoephedrine, phenylpropanolamine, phenylephrine, ephedrine) – avoid 2 weeks
　Cocaine – avoid 2 weeks.
Thyroid block
　I-123 MIBG Lugol's solution – five drops orally 1 h before radiotracer injection, 5 drops same day night and next morning
　I-131 MIBG (treatment) – five drops every day starting 3 days prior the exam and 2 weeks after. (SSKI can also be used).
Dose *Localization:* I-123 MIBG 5–10 mCi/ I-131 MIBG 0.5 mCi. *Treatment* I-131 MIBG 200–400 mCi (treatment as inpatient under radiation safety guidelines).
Prior to treatment with I-131 – IV injection of 1 mCi of Tc-99m pertechnetate or 1 mCi of Tc-99m DTPA to insure line patency.
Image I-123 MIBG – 24 h images. I-131 MIBG – 7–14 days posttreatment.
Critical Organ *I-131 MIBG* Liver *I-123 MIBG* Bladder.
Distribution Liver, adrenal medulla, heart, salivary glands, and spleen (rich adrenergic innervations). 20 % GI tract (free iodine).
Clearance Renal; about 40–50 % within 24 h, 70–90 % within 4 days.

Suggested Reading
- Emilio Bombardieri et al (2010). I-131/I-123-Metaiodobenzylguanidine (mIBG) scintigraphy: procedure guidelines for tumour imaging. Eur J Nucl Med Mol Imaging 37:2436–2446

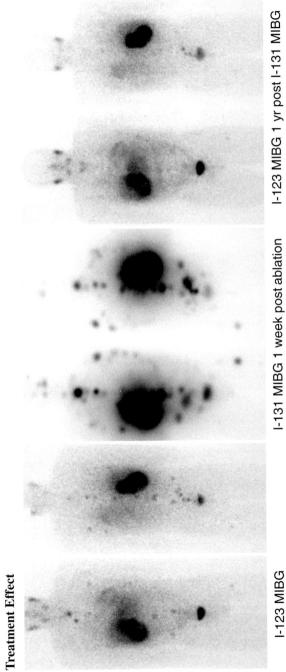

Index

A

Ablation
  bone metastases
    alpha emitter Ra-223 chloride (Xofigo),
      221–222
    beta-minus emitters, 219–220
  liver tumor, radioembolization with
    yttrium-90 microspheres, 216–218
  lymphoma
    bexxar I-131 tositumomab, 223–225
    Y-90 zevalin Y-90 ibritumomab
      tiuxetan, 226–228
  neuroendocrine tumor, I-131 MIBG,
    229–230
  thyroid
    with I-131 NaI. high-dose treatment
      >33 mCi, 211–215
    with I-131 Na. low-dose treatment
      <33 mCi, 210
Alzheimer's disease, 38, 41
Angiotensin-converting enzyme (ACE)
    inhibition renography
  abnormal pattern, 148
  ACE inhibitor, 146
  indication, 146
  interpretation, 147
  protocol, 146–147
  radiopharmaceuticals, 146
  renin-angiotensin system, 146
Annihilation (interaction with β+ particle with
    electron), 8

B

Bladder, 149–151
Bone metastases, palliation of pain
  alpha emitter Ra-223 chloride (Xofigo),
    221–222
  beta-minus emitters, 219–220

Breast
  lymphoscintigraphy
    Tc-99m tilmanocept (lymphoseek),
      83–85
    ultrafiltered Tc-99m sulfur colloid,
      81–82
  Tc-99m sestamibi (MIBI), 77–80
Breast-feeding guidelines, 3
Bremsstrahlung, 9

C

Cell cycle sensitivity, 6
Center of rotation (COR), SPECT, 17
Cerebral death scan
  distribution and clearance, 34
    brain nonspecific agents, 36
    brain-specific agents, 35
  dose, 32
  false negative, 33
  false positive, 33
  mechanism, 32
  negative scan, 32
  poor prognostic signs, 33
  positive scan, 32–33
  target organ, 32
  Tc-99m, 32
  Tc-99m DTPA/Tc-99m
    pertechnetate, 32
  Tc-99m HMPAO/Tc-99m ECD, 32
  tracers, 32
Cerebral perfusion, 37
Ceretec© (Tc-99m HMPAO)
  abnormal distribution, 207
  distribution and clearance,
    204–206
  dose, 204
  indications, 204
  mechanism, 204

© Springer International Publishing Switzerland 2017
B. Savir-Baruch, B.J. Barron, *RadTool Nuclear Medicine Flash Facts*,
DOI 10.1007/978-3-319-24636-9

Printed in the United States
By Bookmasters